FIBROMYALGIA RELIEF:

*A Science-Based Approach
to Healing Body, Mind, and Spirit*

By Lars Clausen

Illustrations by Anne Jacobsen Clausen

www.ICEMethod.com
www.MyFibromyalgiaRelief.com

Copyright © 2013 Lars C. Clausen

All rights reserved

ISBN 9791484135587

"I must be willing to give up what I am in order to become what I will be."
Albert Einstein

Contents

Preface · iix
Introduction · xv

PART ONE

The ICE Method

1 – Enter the Calm State · 21
2 – What Just Happened? · 25
3 - Bring the Calm State to Emotions · 35
4 - Memory Reconsolidation Science · 49
5 – ICE Your Past · 61
6 - Your Peptide Timeline · 71

PART TWO:

Stress

7 - How Long Will It Take? · 81
8 – It's Everywhere · 93
9 – Body, Mind, and Fibromyalgia · 99

PART THREE

Health in a Stress-filled World

    10 – A Brief History of Stress   117

    11 - Attachments and Peptides   129

    12 - Energy and Matter   141

    13 – The ICE Method   153

    Epilogue: A Review   157

    Disclaimer   161

    Notes   163

Preface

Turn off your fight-or-flight response and you will feel better. Your fibromyalgia symptoms may decrease or disappear if you become aware of the state of calm. The paradoxical state of calm allows your body to turn off your fight-or-flight response and enjoy improved health. When your body is calm you produce a chemistry that allows your body to rest and heal. When you are in fight-or-flight mode your body chemistry focuses only on immediate survival. While fight-or-flight helps us survive danger, getting stuck in stress mode causes our health to suffer.

In this book you will learn what I call The ICE Method, based on the latest scientific discoveries of cell biology and neuroscience. A recent neuroscientific discovery called "memory reconsolidation" gives new possibilities for transforming stored emotions in the chemistry of your brain. The acronym ICE stands for *Identify*, *Calm*, and then *Exchange*. I will first show you The ICE Method process to reduce or eliminate your fibromyalgia symptoms. Then I will explain what lies behind the process and why it works. Then you will have a new tool to help you get on with your life.

You could find the information in this book elsewhere. I did. And you can find more experienced facilitators of healing than me. I know a number of them. The reason I write this book is not because I have discovered anything unique. I write because I have combined a number of scientific insights that have allowed many people to experience relief. Millions of people in the United States, and many more around the world, suffer debilitating effects from fibromyalgia. I've experienced success in sharing this method, and I hope it can be effective for you. I would like for people with fibromyalgia to have a simple process for ending their suffering

As fibromyalgia specialist, Dr. Ginevra Liptan has stated in her book, *Figuring Out Fibromyalgia*; "medical science has not yet figured out how to turn off the switch of the stress response that gets stuck in the ON position in fibromyalgia. When we do that we will have found a cure."[1]

Western medical practices typically have rather limited success in treating fibromyalgia. I believe this is because of what Dr. Liptan has noted – that "medical science has not yet figured out how to turn off the switch of the stress response that gets stuck in the ON position." What I can do is to show you a simple way to turn down your fight-or-flight response. Turn off your fight-or-flight stress response and you can begin to feel

Preface

better. My goal and my wish are for you and for everyone who has fibromyalgia to learn how easily you can turn off your fight-or-flight response.

During the past few years I have worked with over one hundred people, including a study in a fibromyalgia clinic with 39 patients suffering severe symptoms. I have been amazed to see how easily one can reduce or eliminate pain. As easy as this process is, and as much as people enjoy the feeling of calm, I also see how often people get stuck back in their old familiar stress state.

Recently, I helped a man use The ICE Method to completely eliminate his sciatica back pain symptoms during his first session. He said he'd use The ICE Method "all the time," he was so amazed by his pain going away. A week later, he called to say he was too busy for his second appointment, and yes, his back was hurting again. For the relief of pain, one must continue turning off the fight-or-flight response until it no longer stays stuck in the ON position. In this book I will show you how to do this. Once you know the process, you will have a tool for relieving your flight-or-flight response patterns whenever they arise.

Entering the calm state can often provide healing for body, mind, and spirit. As I will explain, most of what we react to in our daily lives can't actually physically hurt us (the overdue bill, the cranky boss, the whiny kids). We don't really need our body to go into fight-or-flight mode to respond to these situations. Fight-or-flight only truly needs to engage during a clear present physical danger (the proverbial tiger, or a bus about to run you over in a crosswalk). Unfortunately, most of us have learned to respond to overdue bills and other anxieties with the same fight-or-flight chemistry as when a real tiger attacks.

Far more than necessary, we live in an anxious state, yet in reality we face very few immediate physical threats that might cause us bodily harm. We actually don't need our fight-or-flight response turned on except for the rare immediate physical threat. If we could figure out how to turn off the fight-or-flight response, we would discover that it's almost always safe for our body chemistry to be calm. My goal is to show you how to do this.

If you feel ready to explore how calm can change your life, then this book could well provide a life-changing addition to your daily experience. As you learn to bring this calm to your life, you can enjoy healing for mind, body, and spirit. As you learn to live your life from the calm state, then you will bring greater peace to your life. I wrote this book for you who wish to have calm as the ground state of your life.

I also understand that it takes an effort to try "one more thing." If you're like most, you've already tried many alternatives for finding relief of your fibromyalgia symptoms. It takes energy and courage to risk once more in the possibility of a solution to your problems. I hope that this approach which honors body, mind, and spirit together, will engage your attention.

Preface

On the other hand, if this approach doesn't make sense for where you are in your journey, that's okay too. I trust you will respect what you feel is best for you. If *Fibromyalgia Relief* doesn't feel right at this time, perhaps you will want to find a place on your shelf to let this book rest awhile. Maybe sometime in the future you'll find it worthwhile to take another look at this process for turning off your fight-or-flight stress response to reduce or eliminate fibromyalgia symptoms. If, though, you're ready to turn off your fight-or-flight stress response now and start living from the calm state, then let's get started.

Two notes before we begin:

First, if your memories are particularly traumatic; if you "dissociate" from the memories when you become aware of them, or if you have severe anxiety when you become aware of past situations in your life, then you may benefit by having a skilled person assist you in this process. Please visit MyFibromyalgiaRelief.com for helpful resources. Consult a professional psychologist or medical caregiver if you have questions.

Second, I am not a doctor. I have a Master's degree in Mechanical Engineering and I earned a Master of Divinity degree to become a pastor. I also hold a Guinness World record from unicycling through all fifty states. I work to facilitate healing, and my goal is to help people enjoy better emotional, spiritual, and physical health. Read my disclaimer at the back of this book. You must take responsibility for whatever you adopt from this book.

My best wishes to you,

Lars Clausen

Introduction

If you're suffering from fibromyalgia symptoms right now, I recommend going to Chapter One immediately. This chapter begins directly with instructions for entering the calm state.

Chapter Three and Chapter Five provide the remainder of the simple instructions for using The ICE Method. You can read only these three chapters of this book and begin using the method now.

After each of the three chapters on how to do The ICE Method, I've included a chapter explaining my understanding of the science of each part of The ICE Method. I've included these chapters because I believe understanding what informs this process will increase your confidence in the method and its results. I've come to trust The ICE Method completely for my own life and for the people I work with, partly because I see the results, and partly because there's scientific research that I believe is consistent with the healing that I see people experience.

A trusted doctor friend of mine reviewed *Fibromyalgia Relief* and suggested I clarify how I use the scientific findings quoted in this book. The research I've studied has helped me create The ICE Method, but it does not prove the mechanisms for why The ICE Method works. Nor does the research prove that I'm correct in my understanding of how fibromyalgia symptoms can be relieved. What the research findings have done is to help me creatively develop my practice – "if the brain or the body shows this result in an experiment, then maybe I could do this in a session and get a good result." I believe that what I'm presenting in this book is consistent with available scientific findings, but it's important to clarify that current research does not prove how The ICE Method achieves results. So, thanks to the science for inspiration, and thanks to the clients and the experience for coming up with a process that works. *Fibromyalgia Relief* is my current best understanding of a process that has resulted in healing for many people.

In Part Two of *Fibromyalgia Relief* I hope to demonstrate the benefits of making The ICE Method an ongoing part of your life. In Part Two I want to give you a better feel for some of the science findings about fibromyalgia. Chronic stress affects our body and every part of our being, which explains part of why the calm state can provide such relief of fibromyalgia symptoms. I also want to provide some examples of memory reconsolidation and how it happens in places other than The ICE Method.

Finally, in Part Three, I want to invite you on a journey that may surprise you in a book about fibromyalgia. If you're interested in healing, and if you understand that chronic stress has such an impact on our lives, then you also might start asking some of the same questions as me;

- Why is our world such a stressful place to live in?"

- Was our world always like this?

- Is there a better way than 'survival of the fittest'?

Part of my personal experience includes living in a hunting-gathering culture in Nome, Alaska. There I watched and learned that traditional societies based their survival on cooperation rather than competition. And now our most modern science, quantum physics, takes us away from survival of the fittest toward an intensely cooperative understanding of the universe.

You might not have expected such topics included alongside of fibromyalgia, but once you've learned The ICE Method, I invite you to enter into my conversation with these concepts. Shutting off our fight-or-flight response is key to reducing or eliminating the symptoms of fibromyalgia. When we look for the causes of stress in our personal lives, we end up looking at what causes stress in our world.

Chapter One. Chapter Three. Chapter Five. Start with these and see if the steps of The ICE Method provide you relief from your symptoms. Then enjoy the rest of the book depending on your interests. Whatever you use, I hope you find the information helpful.

In this book you'll read examples from some of the people I have worked with. No names are provided, and identifying details have been changed to maintain anonymity. I work with people with many different types of emotional and physical pain. I'll include some examples of people with symptoms other than fibromyalgia so you can see that The ICE Method can be used for more than just your fibromyalgia symptoms.

Once again, before you begin, remember you must take personal responsibility for whatever you choose to use. I am not a doctor. Read the disclaimer in the appendix. If you have questions, see your doctor or your mental health care provider.

PART ONE

The ICE Method

1 – Enter the Calm State

This process will allow you to turn off your fight-or-flight stress response Most people feel both physical and emotional relief when they enter a calm state. Here's how to do it.

Pick a point on a wall and just watch that point. It could be a doorknob, a corner of a painting, the top of a tree or whatever. Just watch the point for a moment. If your mind gets pulled away from observing the point, no problem. As soon as you notice, bring your attention back to the point.

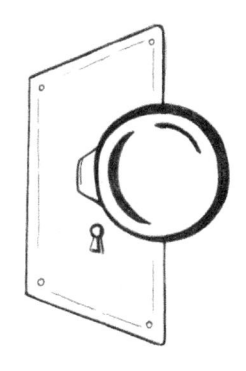

What happens in this moment of attention affects the chemistry of your mind and your body. Whatever your mind pays attention to, your body always follows. Like when you get angry, you can feel the tension rise in your body. Your body prepares automatically to respond to what made you angry.

When you observe this single point, because it's so simple, your body has very little to be responsible for.

You may or may not feel it, but your body will automatically start to relax a bit. You may feel your breath beginning to slow. This is a very important point. The body has little to do when the mind observes only a single point. As you observe the single point you become less reactive to your external environment and the chemistry of your body will begin to change. This is the first of three steps in beginning to let your mind lead your body to a calm and healing place.

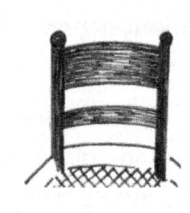

Now choose a second point and observe it. It should be easy to see both the first point and this second point without having to move your head. Your mind will calm and your body will relax a little bit more, because looking at this point is once again such a simple task for your mind. When your mind focuses on something simple then your body has very little to react against. Body follows mind.

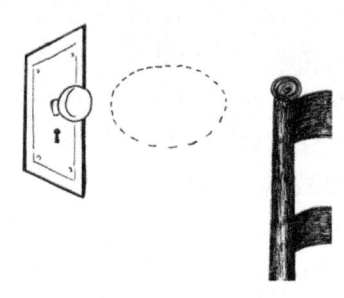

Excellent, now the third step involves shifting your attention and observing the empty space that lies between your two points. Behind the points you may see the wall or a mountain or whatever fills the background. But

Enter The Calm State

between the two points you can visualize the empty space, the space between the two points that has nothing in it. Observe that space.

This empty space has nothing in it to see or sense. When you observe the empty space with your mind, you observe nothing. When you observe nothing with your mind, you signal your body it has nothing it needs to react to in the outside environment. Your body gets the signal that it can move completely into rest mode. I call this your calm state, and you will find it extraordinarily beneficial for your health.

Most people describe the feeling of the calm space as "delicious." I agree. When you have your mind observe this space with nothing in it, you actually give the 50-100 trillion cells of your body the signal that your outside environment is completely safe and free of immediate physical threat.

When this happens you have turned off your fight-or-flight response.

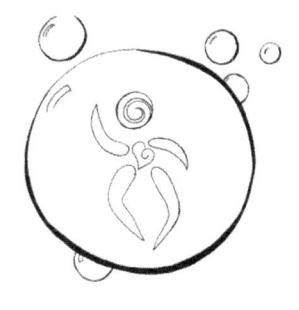

The important thing about giving your body this signal of complete safety is that for whatever time you experience this space, your body has nothing to react to in the outside world. When you're in this calm state your body turns naturally and fully towards tending your internal needs.[2] Important chemical and biological changes happen when you're in this state – all good healing stuff.

I'll explain later how I understand the science of the calm space – for now, just enjoy being in this refreshing calm state as often as you can, and for as long as you find time. Most people with fibromyalgia have a lot of stress in their lives. A lot of other people have a lot of stress, too. Calm is helpful for anyone with stress. Let yourself be aware of the calm space. You will feel better.

2 – What Just Happened?

You just had a conscious experience of having your body follow your mind. This book exists to show you how helpful this can be for your health. For most people I work with, entering the calm state is the most important part of healing. When you gain conscious awareness of your mind, your fight-or-flight mechanism can shut off and your body can drop into rest mode. Here's how this works.

For almost everyone, the calm state feels like a revelation. Most of us have lived our lives thinking our bodies control our physical health. We believe genes or food or exercise or medicines or surgeries determine our health. We believe physical interventions control our physical well-being. We spend our lives reacting to flu bugs, toothaches, joint pain, and much more. If we have fibromyalgia most of us believe we have few options other than a physical reaction to the physical symptoms, either with medicine or with changes in our lifestyle. If we shift to understanding fibromyalgia in the following way, then the possibilities for healing grow tremendously:

1. The cells of our body respond to stress, and fibromyalgia symptoms are affected by stress.

2. If stress continues, the chemical results can begin impacting the function of the body. The symptoms of fibromyalgia can result, including: joint pain, inflammation, insomnia, skin sensitivity, irritable bowel, brain fog, etc.

3. Chronic stress can put the body in a stuck response state where our physical systems are perpetually out of whack.

4. Calming the mind calms the body, turns off the fight-or-flight response and relieves the body. In many cases, when this happens we feel better.

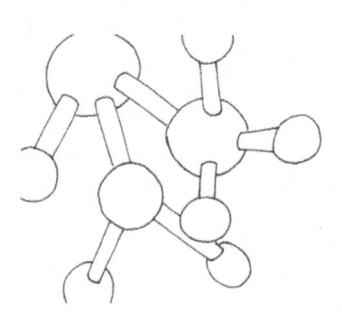

I'll provide more about the research that's inspired me about stress, fight-or-flight, and the function of the body in Chapter Nine. It turns out that our emotions and the chemistry of our bodies have a direct connection through a molecule called a peptide.[3] A peptide consists of amino acid molecules. Different arrangements of amino acids create different peptides. If you imagine that the amino acids are like Lego pieces, then the different peptides are like differing combinations of Lego blocks stacked together. Every time you experience an emotion, at that very instant you create a peptide that corresponds to that emotion.

For example, when you experience anger, you create one combination of amino acids. When you experience sadness or fear, happiness or contentment, you create other peptides. (Thanks to Candace Pert for bringing this knowledge to the public in her 1997 book, *Molecules of Emotion*. There are hundreds of different types of peptides and there is a whole field of medical research devoted to peptides: psychoneuroimmunology. For this book, I'm going to keep things simple and use the general term "peptide." If you want more detail, you will find lots to explore.)[4]

These peptides you create provide the instructions to every one of the 50-100 trillion cells of your body for what each cell should do. You can feel this happening as soon as you pay attention to your emotions. Feel the tenseness in your body as you experience anger or fear. Feel the reaction in your body when a deep sadness overcomes you. Feel the relaxation arising in a moment of contentment. A bit more on the peptide system, and then we'll explore what happens physically when you open up your awareness of the calm state.

This peptide system provides an amazing connection between our mind, our body and the environment around us. If you become aware of this connection and you begin using this awareness, your life will change immensely.

If a bus is barreling toward you, you will experience fear and you will automatically jump out of the way. Thank you fear peptide! This example shows what the fight-or-flight part of the peptide system was designed for, to keep you in a healthy relationship with your environment. When a fear or anger emotion arises it happens because your fight-or-flight response got activated.

In a normal situation, after the dangerous bus passes by your fight-or-flight system would shut back down and you would quickly return to a relaxed state. In long ago days when threats were tigers and such, many researchers believe that relaxation happened naturally after the threat ended. If you survived the tiger, your fight-or-flight system would settle back down and you'd return to lounging under the shade of the fruit tree.

In these modern times, though, stresses pile up so persistently for most people, and with such intensity, that most of us end up with some degree of constant fight-or-flight activation. We worry about events in the future. We feel emotions about memories from the past.

When I explain this to people with fibromyalgia, the majority nod their head and say, "That's me. I have a lot of anxiety." A good number also have a strong perfectionism, which can create even more stress.

For some of us, then, our stress response eventually gets stuck in the ON position. At this point, our body experiences a constant stress, a constant activation of the fight-or-flight stress response. Instead of resting and restoring our body, we become ever more weary, exhausted, painful, and symptomatic. The immune system and other functions of the body end up out of whack, creating inflammation and various reactions in the body. For some of us this stuck fight-or-flight response eventually shows up as fibromyalgia. For others the symptoms show up differently. For any person who experiences stress, this calm state exercise will provide health benefits.

Let's look at what happens when you open yourself to the awareness of your calm state. Remember that at every moment, your mind-body is creating a peptide to match your emotion and that these peptides direct the activity of all your cells.

If you carry around chronic stress your cells receive the instruction to ALWAYS be on guard and ready to defend against threats from your environment.

When you observe the first point with your mind, you make a conscious intervention in whatever's going on and you direct your mind to focus its attention on something simple and something specific. By making this simple conscious intervention you take your mind away from whatever pressing concerns are causing your stress. Because focusing on the single item is so simple and so non-emotional, you start creating a calm peptide that matches this relaxed state. You will feel the subtle sensation of your body beginning to relax.

Since the points you observe exist out in your external environment, your emotion still has an external reference. As long as the points exist outside of you, you continue responding to your outside world. By focusing on the second point we create the space between the two points, the empty space where nothing exists. When the mind observes nothing in the outside world, then the mind creates a peptide to match this state of complete emotional calm. The peptide instruction to all the cells of the body is, "relax, there's nothing in the outside world that our body cells need to react to."

I feel thankful to Frank Kinslow for sharing the two-point exercise in his 2008 book, *The Secret of Instant Healing*.[5] Meditational calming practices are common and varied, and other practices might work equally well. I like the two-point method because it's so simple and it works for people, virtually without fail. I also prefer the two-point method and the empty space in between because it provides such a strong visual image for what happens in our body when we experience calm. When this calming practice combines with Candace Pert's contributions about emotions and peptides the result offers a powerful opportunity for creating better health.

When the mind observes this space with nothing in it, then the mind receives a signal that holds no danger. When the mind observes nothing in the outside world, when the mind senses no danger, then the body has no reaction. A calm peptides forms and then permeates the body with instructions for each of the trillions of cells of the body. The fight-or-flight mechanism turns off. The incessant pressure that has created body system disorder suddenly stops. The body relaxes. In this mode your cells actually turn from an external response mode to a complete focus on internal cellular healing, rest, and restoration. (Thanks to Bruce Lipton for his very readable book on how this works on a cellular level, *The Biology of Belief*.)[6]

When we are in a rest state, the cell membranes switch to open growth mode. In growth mode cells can begin communicating with each other. This calm state is different from when your body reacts to stress. Under stress the cell wall closes off and goes into protection mode. In protection mode your cells stop metabolizing energy and eliminating waste through the cell membrane. Other important functions stop as well. Your body quits focusing on long term health and shifts to protecting you from immediate threats. Protection mode helps you survive immediate danger, but you're not supposed to be in protection mode all the time. If your cells get stuck in protection mode you compromise your long term health.

If you live with constant stress, your body must spend part of its energy protecting against perceived threats. Less energy remains for maintaining and restoring your physical health. When you use The ICE Method or some other technique, your mind will calm and your cell membranes open. Then your body's information system can discover needs and your cells can begin cooperating internally. The body can create more chemicals of healing and more restorative medicines than pharmaceutical companies have ever discovered. When the body rests in the calm state, then your internal pharmacy kicks in and immediately begins to produce the chemistry of health. This is our natural state. We only need to get out of the way. Because of this natural restoration that starts when the mind becomes calm, fibromyalgia pain often begins diminishing and sometimes disappears completely.

The relationship between calm and healing works because the body always follows the mind.

When you use the mind to interrupt and stop the stress response, the body's natural healing capacity is free to work fully on behalf of our health and well-being.

As I said at the beginning of Chapter One – the more time you spend in the calm state, the better your life will feel. In the next chapters I want to address two further expansions on the calm state that will make the calm space an even more powerful tool for you,

The first expansion involves how to deal directly with non-calm emotions as they arise. When you learn this you can quickly return to the calm state and restore your cells to their functions of healing, rest, and restoration.

The second elaboration shows a method that allows you to calm past memories, even including early memories of trauma. The technique is simple, based on a scientific discovery called *memory reconsolidation*.[7] This laboratory discovery, made only in 2004, has not yet made its way into most therapies. I believe that it will someday be a foundation of most effective therapies because memory reconsolidation can actually replace the stored emotional peptides in old memories with new emotional peptides of calm and peace. The content of the memory remains, but the old emotional charge from the memory gets replaced with a peaceful emotion. As I promised at the beginning of this book, I will explain how I understand the science of the process in Chapter 4 after I share the technique.

When we get to dealing with past emotions and even past traumas, I want you to pay attention to your needs. If you dissociate from your memories or if you experience strong reactions, you may want professional care, perhaps a professional therapist, or your medical doctor. Be gentle with yourself. As you'll discover when you continue reading, The ICE Method process offers you a completely calm approach to bringing peace into your present as well as your past experiences.

3 - Bring the Calm State to Emotions

I will make a guess - few people ask you what actual emotion you feel about living with fibromyalgia. Sometimes when I ask about the emotion, people can't immediately name what they feel about fibromyalgia. I want to ask you this question now. And I want to invite you to give whatever time it takes to feel the emotion when you ask yourself what it feels like to live with fibromyalgia.

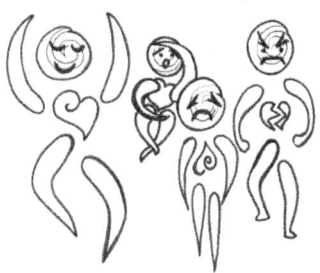

No better or worse emotions exist about having fibromyalgia, but knowing which emotions you feel will make a big difference for your health. Experiencing this emotion will take you out of the calm space for a moment. Don't worry; we'll get back to calm again in just a bit. For now, take a few moments and allow yourself to feel your emotion about living with fibromyalgia. We don't have to analyze or figure out why you feel this emotion, we just need to discover it and let ourselves feel it for a brief moment.

Some people feel angry about their fibromyalgia. No wonder. Some people feel afraid of their fibromyalgia. No surprise. Others feel sad. That too is common. Take this moment to let yourself access whatever emotion or emotions you hold about living with fibromyalgia.

Notice that if you describe your emotion as "frustration," or "irritation," these give you a gentler way of verbalizing the basic emotion, anger. You might describe your feeling as "anxious." That's okay, but I want you to see that anxiety is a less potent way of describing the emotion of fear.

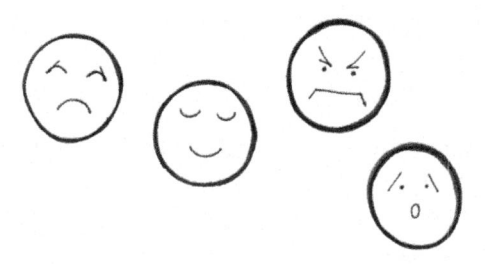

If possible, let yourself feel the most basic possible emotion about your fibromyalgia. You may have more than one of these three – anger, sadness, fear - take the first one that comes up. If none of these seem to fit, take whatever word best describes your emotion about living with fibromyalgia. The process can start with whatever you identify.

Again, I'll explain the science later; for now let's do the process. I want you to really experience at a gut level what your identified emotion does in your body.

Whatever emotion you hold about living with fibromyalgia, that emotion in your mind also provides constant physical instructions for your physical body. Anger or fear will result in chronic tension. Sadness will stress your system. Your bodily systems will end up over-engaged by these feelings. Your symptoms will almost certainly escalate.

One woman I worked with insisted she had no emotion about living with her fibromyalgia. When I gently asked if she ever felt anger, she replied, "Never. That doesn't do any good. If I ever let myself feel anger I hurt so bad I have to sit in my recliner with a heating blanket and turn off all the lights in the room."

In the remainder of the session with this woman I tried as carefully as possible to help her become aware of the connection between emotions, peptides, and the function of our body. Whenever I mentioned emotion, she seemed to shut the words out.

Know this. Your body follows your mind.

Your mind always creates peptides that correspond to your emotions. If you can stay with me here, I want to show you a process to calm whatever emotion or emotions you have about living with fibromyalgia.

We're going to change the emotional peptide you have stored in connection with your emotion about living with fibromyalgia. When we change the peptide we change the instruction to your body. We learned this in Chapter One by going into the calm state. Now we're going to learn to use this calm state to actually go in and change the emotional peptides stored in your brain.

As soon as you identified your emotion about your fibromyalgia you created the possibility of replacing that emotion with calm. You can literally exchange the stored emotional peptide with a calm peptide. Scientists have named this process *memory reconsolidation*. I'll explain the science later, but let's experience it first.

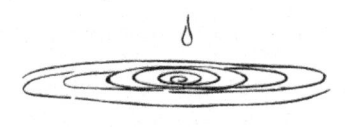

To replace your angry, sad, fearful or other identified emotion about living with fibromyalgia, we have to step back from the emotion you just identified and return to the calm state. If the emotion turns out to be intense, then choosing calm will not feel like an obvious choice. This is, though, the choice that needs to be made.

Instead of continuing to react to the emotion, use the calm process and return to a state of calm.

We described this calm state process in Chapter One. First choose a single point and observe it. This simple focus of the mind starts to calm the body. Next choose a second point and observe it. Finally, observe the space in between the two points and allow yourself to become aware of the calm space. The mind gives the

Bring the Calm State to Emotions

body the signal that there's nothing requiring a fight-or-flight response. The body can enter rest mode. Go back to Chapter One if you want to review.

As you become aware of the calm space again, you'll notice that feeling of relaxation and peace returning. This will happen even though just a moment before you were feeling the emotion that you hold about living with fibromyalgia. As soon as you're back in the calm state, peptide molecules of emotional calm begin flowing throughout your body. These calm peptides immediately head out to all the cells of your body and return you to a state of healing and rest. This is what we did in Chapter One.

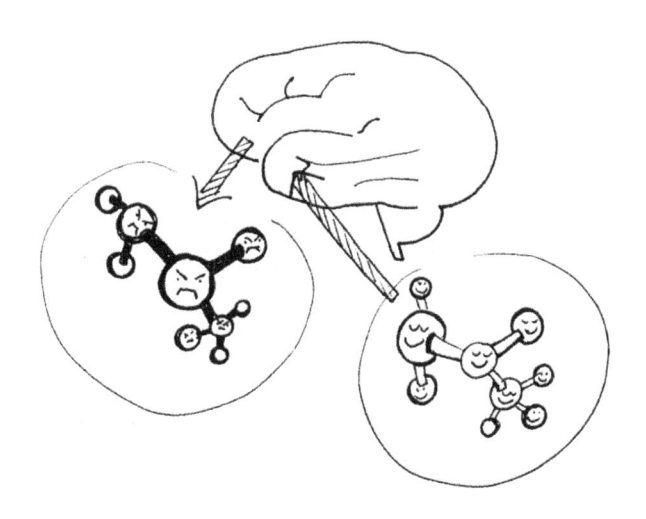

Now we will experience a further way of consciously using these calm molecules. According to the discovery of memory reconsolidation, these calm peptides can actually replace the emotional peptides that store your feeling about fibromyalgia. Give yourself a few moments in this calm state and then I'll explain.

In the calm state, I imagine the calm molecules going out to all the cells of my body. I also imagine filling up a bucket until it overflows with calm peptide molecules. We'll use that bucket of calm peptides to calm your emotions about living with fibromyalgia.

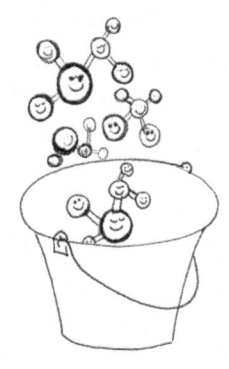

All you need to do now is to move from observing the calm state back to observing your identified emotion about fibromyalgia. As you observe your emotion about fibromyalgia again you literally bring the calm peptides back to the brain cells that have stored your emotion about fibromyalgia. The remarkable science piece discovered in 2004 showed in a laboratory setting that when you activate a memory, the emotions stored with the memories also become active. The old emotion can then exchange with a new emotional peptide. This happens when you bring a new emotional feeling (calm) to the old state (for example; anger, sadness, or fear). More later on the science, but at this point I would like for you to experience the process.

First, observe the emotion that you just identified about living with fibromyalgia. As you go back from the calm space to observe the original emotion, you automatically bring the state of calm to replace the emotion of that old memory.

What did you feel? One of two possibilities will arise. One possibility is that you will feel calm now about being a person who has fibromyalgia. In that case, you're all set, you have discharged an emotion that has been adding chronic stress to your body, throwing your physical system out of whack, and giving you pain.

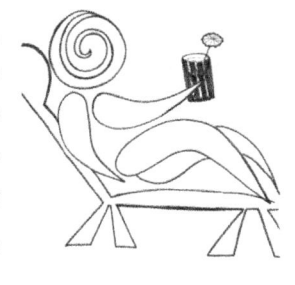

The other possibility is that after you do this first round of exchanging the peptides you have about fibromyalgia, something else shows up, another layer of emotion. If this happens then you can repeat the process with whatever you have newly become aware of. Perhaps you felt anger first, and now you feel sadness. Or perhaps you first felt anger about all the pain, and now you feel anger about the things you miss out on because of your fibromyalgia. Whatever it is, identify the new feeling, the new memory, the new physical sensation, whatever shows up. Just as you identified your first emotion about having fibromyalgia, once that reconsolidates, you can observe whatever shows up next. Do the calm process again, and then go back to observe the non-calm emotion. Repeat this process, back and forth, until you get through the layers and all that remains is calm.

When I work with people with fibromyalgia and when we pay attention to their emotions about their disease, we don't focus at all on their physical pain during this time. The emotions vary, but as long as the emotions get activated, they can replace with calm. Sometimes pain disappears in fifteen minutes. Sometimes the process takes a number of hour-long sessions, unlayering the emotions and experiences piece by piece.

One woman I worked with had loved her high-pressure on-call work as an emergency medical technician. After work she pushed on to other activities such that she slept only a few hours each night. After her fibromyalgia began causing severe pain in her joints, she was reduced to only the most absolutely necessary movements.

The emotion this woman identified was strong anger about all the activities she could no longer participate in. After identifying her anger and going back and forth between the calm space she noticeably relaxed. Her spouse was present during the session and he remarked that he hadn't seen his wife so relaxed since her fibromyalgia had started three years before. During the session this woman's joint pain dropped to only a faint irritation. "Look, she said, I can move my fingers and they don't hurt."

All we had focused on was the emotion she held about having fibromyalgia. In the process of exchanging those angry peptides with calm peptides, this woman's body began to react with much less pain.

In Chapter Seven I will address how long it may take you to get well. The process for this woman would simply be to continue observing whatever does not feel calm in her life and exchanging emotional peptides.

I have been doing The ICE Method process for myself for over a year now, and after the first few weeks of using this process I realized I was spending more and more of my time in the calm state. Now only infrequently do non-calm emotions upset me, but when they do I pull out this calming process and use it right away. At this point I know I have a choice. Either I can react to emotionally charged peptides that will create a physical effect in my body, or I can create calm for my mind and my body. I have grown to recognize that this calm state creates much better health for me. I have also grown to completely trust this peptide exchange process for myself and those I work with.

I now use The ICE Method for almost everything. The other day I got a call from my dentist to tell me I was late, my appointment time had started five minutes earlier. As I hurried into my car and started the fifteen minute drive to the dentist, I soon became aware I was in fight-or-flight mode. My body had tightened, I could feel the tension across my chest and back — my hands were clenched on the steering wheel. As soon as I became aware of this I also became aware that missing the appointment was upsetting and embarrasing, but not an actual threat to my physical well-being. Once I became aware that I didn't need a bodily fight-or-flight response to deal with being late I found two points on the dashboard of the car and then returned to the calm space. I arrived at the dentist feeling calm about whatever might happen, either the dentist adjusting her schedule or me rescheduling the appointment. After the initial fight-or-flight response, I quickly returned to a calm healing mode for my body. I use The ICE Method all the time, because it works for the big issues in life as well as the everyday bumps in the road. My health is better because of The ICE Method. I worry less. I sleep better. I have more energy.

A quick note about our good memories and the satisfying emotions of joy, peace, and happiness. An extroverted friend once asked me if this calming process was going to turn her into a quiet introvert! It could perhaps, but only if that's what a person wanted. The purpose of The ICE Method is to deal with the distress that impacts our emotional and physical health. The ICE Method allows our body to remain in a healthy rest state, but we can still actively engage with our surroundings. We can keep all the satisfying emotions of our life unchanged and just deal with the distress. We can remain extroverted or introverted, if that is our wish.

The woman who earlier told me she had to retreat to her easy chair if she ever felt anger never returned for a second session. In fact, she emailed me to tell me

Bring the Calm State to Emotions

I had come "dangerously close to telling her that her fibromyalgia was all in her head."

I think I have some understanding of where this woman is coming from. Way too much blame and accusation has been thrown around in the past about the disease of fibromyalgia. This book holds no blame and no judgment. There is no blame and no judgment in the process of memory reconsolidation. Memory reconsolidation happens for every human being whether we have fibromyalgia or perfect health. It's a chemical process of peptides in our brains and bodies. Every one of us stores experiences and emotions in the synapses and neurons of our brains. Understanding memory reconsolidation gives us the opportunity to calm old emotions, change the peptide signals to our body, and experience emotional and physical relief.

For the woman who took refuge in her heating blanket, as long as she continues to store those peptides of anger in her brain cell synapses, she will likely continue to experience painful physical reactions to her emotions of anger. As long as any of us store non-calm emotional peptides, we will live in reaction to those peptides. When we discover that we feel ready to have those emotions become calm – this process will be waiting. As we remove our emotional reactivity, we can increase the freedom in our lives.

I'll share more about process details later, but for now just be aware you can have layers of emotion built up, and you can deal with all of them, one by one. As one emotion becomes calm, then the mind may become aware of a next layer. Simply continue the process of going back and forth between observing the calm state and observing whatever emotion you identify.

There's no set number of steps in this process, and there's no hurry either. Know that every time you replace a disturbing emotional peptide with a calm one, you are relieving stress on your body and ultimately you will feel better.

When your mind sends calm signals to your body, you feel better than when messages of anger or fear or sadness cause chronic stress in your body.

As I said in Chapter One, the more time you spend in the calm state, the better you will feel. Now in Chapter Three you have discovered a way to calm past emotions that would otherwise cause chronic stress to your body. When you have emotions that do not feel calm, your body reacts with some amount of fight-or-flight response. This takes energy. Calm, on the other hand, provides healing, rest, and restoration.

My suggestion – make the calm state your default state. Stay in this calm state as often as you can. Whenever you notice you have left the calm state, identify the agitating emotion and replace it with calm. Use this process and you will feel better.

Time now for the science of memory reconsolidation. After this next chapter we will return to technique again. I call this full process, The ICE

Method. ICE stands for Identify, Calm, and Exchange. In Chapter Five I will share how The ICE Method lets you use the memory reconsolidation phenomenon to actually calm the memories of your past, even including issues of serious trauma.

4 - Memory Reconsolidation Science

An important discovery occurred in 2004 – we can replace the emotional component of even old memories and eliminate the charge stored in those memories.[8] Scientists call this process *memory reconsolidation*. This discovery has just barely begun to impact the way we work with memory and life. I believe the impact on our understanding of health and the way we provide healthcare will prove enormous.

The traditional understanding in psychology and neuroscience has believed that emotional memories stay fixed in our brains for as long as we live. As psychologist Bruce Ecker explains in *Unlocking The Emotional Brain*, "Before 2000, based on nearly a century of research, neuroscientists believed that the brain did not possess the capability of erasing an existing, established emotional learning from memory."[9]

If we believe emotional learning is fixed, then we have two choices:

1. We may react to our fixed memories by repeating the same actions over and over again.

2. We may work to develop new habits that allow us to respond differently.

Either way, we are stuck reacting to the fixed emotions and events of our memories. Psychologists call the whole range of developing new habits – counteractive therapy.[10]

One way I explain this to clients is to imagine our life as an obstacle course of emotions and events. In certain situations I'll use the word "minefield" because it's vitally important to understand that most of our life is lived reactively, as a reaction to the stored emotions of the past or the emotional concerns of the future. This obstacle course, or minefield, is filled with our emotional reactions to parents, siblings, teachers, and all the other events of our life. In this obstacle course of our life, we have both safe places and dangerous places. We're attracted to the safe places (the good memories) and we're repelled by the dangerous places (the traumas of our past).

The prevailing understanding is that the obstacles of our emotional life are pretty much fixed, just like a real obstacle course has unchangeable features in its design. If we've learned to navigate the course well, then we have a "successful" life. If we don't navigate it well, we find that we keep getting stuck and getting knocked off course. When we go to a therapist or seek other help to become more successful at navigating our life, we are typically trying to create a new habit so we can better navigate through the obstacles. Either way, whether we feel successful or we're trying to develop better habits, we are still *reacting* to the emotional history of our life.

Now science has discovered a powerful new understanding of our emotional life – the obstacles on the course can be completely removed. Instead of the hard work of developing new habits to react to our old fixed patterns, we can replace the charged emotions that have caused us to react. The emotional part of our memories can be replaced using this mechanism of memory reconsolidation. Memory reconsolidation is physically different from what happens when your brain builds a new habit. Creating new habits relies on actually building new neural networks: wiring up new pathways between brain cells.

Instead of creating a counteractive alternative, (a new habit) memory reconsolidation relies on emotions of calm physically replacing old emotional peptides that have caused us fear or anger or sadness, maybe even since childhood. When we do this we eliminate the stress we've been reacting to. Once the old emotional peptide has been replaced with calm, we can choose our action freely instead of reacting to old charged emotions. I have based The ICE Method on this discovery. Here's my understanding of the science of the process.

As I explained earlier, every time you experience an emotion you create a matching peptide. (Brain scientists debate whether the peptide or the emotion happens first, but either way, the order doesn't affect this discovery about memory reconsolidation). You have already seen how emotional peptides provide instructions to your body. For example, if you feel afraid, your body will experience the urge to flee. The peptide also has another function. Peptides literally participate in gluing memories together.

Let's say your emotion of fear gets triggered, because your car gets rear-ended. Along with this emotion, many brain cells will begin connecting so you can create a memory of this car crash. Brain cells have tiny threadlike structures all over them, and these threads create the brain's wiring. The place where the wires connect is called a synapse. Memory reconsolidation occurs at these synapses.

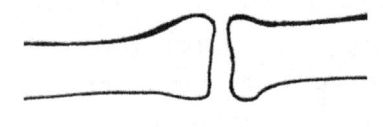

For a memory to form, and for the memory to stick, the synapses must connect and then remain connected – they must somehow glue together. It turns out that the same peptide that gets created from your emotion not only instructs your physical body, it also glues synapses together. At the same time the peptides instruct your body function during an event they also glue your memory together so you can remember the event.

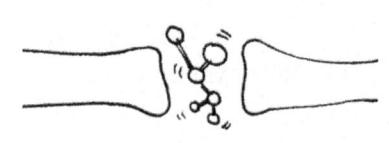

Both body and mind depend on emotional peptides.

You can imagine that your brain cells contain the *content* of your memory (the color of the car that hit you, where the accident occurred, etc.). The synapses contain the *emotion* of the memory (terror, anger, whatever.)

How can the emotions of a memory be switched? First, it turns out when you recall a memory the peptide that glues the synapses together becomes "labile" in the words of the neuroscientists, "fragile" in my words. Basically, this means that the memory becomes activated by your paying attention to it. Memory reconsolidation can only happen on a memory you specifically activate. You can feel thankful for this. You don't have to worry about any sort of full disk reformatting of your brain occurring when you use memory reconsolidation.

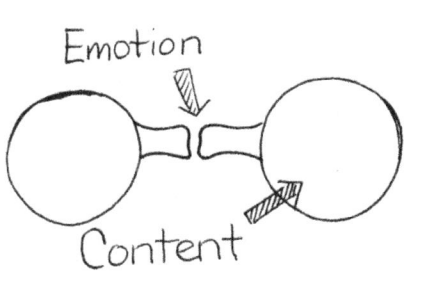

Recalling, or "activating" a memory initiates the reconsolidating process. Scientists have discovered that the memory stays activated for something like six hours, the "window of opportunity." Next, once you activate a memory it turns out that in the synapse, the old emotional peptide must replace with a new peptide molecule.

This is the profound discovery, that the old emotional peptide can be replaced with a different peptide carrying a different emotion.. Let me explain how memory reconsolidation happens normally, without a conscious intervention. Then I'll show you the difference you can experience when you reconsolidate a memory using a conscious intervention such as The ICE Method.

In your normal everyday life, when you recall that car crash memory, you activate the memory. If you pay attention you will feel that original terror emotion rise up again, the same emotion you felt when you got rear-ended. This emotional peptide molecule that corresponds to your feeling about the car crash has now entered a fragile state. It will remain activated for about six hours. Unless you make a conscious intervention, the following chemical process unfolds unconsciously and automatically.

Activate memory:

When you feel the terror from the memory of the car crash, the experience of feeling this emotion causes you to create more new fear peptides again.

Create new peptides:

These newly formed fear peptides are identical to the old fear peptides. Why? Because the same emotion of fear has surfaced again. Feel the same emotion – create the same peptide.

Memory Reconsolidation Science

Body response:

As we learned earlier, peptides instruct our bodies and glue our memories. This is why your body responds to a memory with the same sensations as the actual event, the chemistry is the same. In the example of remembering the car crash, this explains why your body tenses up again.

Reconsolidate memory:

Peptides glue or reglue memories. In this case, the peptides will reglue the synapses from the car crash memory you just activated. The newly formed peptide actually does replace the original peptide. But since the new peptide and the old peptide have the same structure, the emotion feels the same.

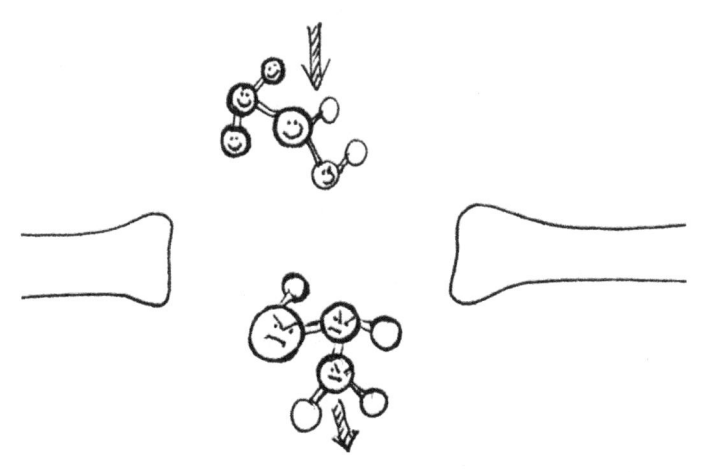

This example shows how memory reconsolidation takes place every time we activate a memory. Most of the time, without a conscious intervention, we just reconsolidate the old memory with more of the original emotion. Even though memory reconsolidation actually happens every time a memory is activated, since no conscious intervention occurs, the terror emotion of the car crash feels permanent.

With this example, you can start to see why early life traumas such as abuse, or later traumas such as war atrocities, rape, or disasters can impact our body and mind so profoundly. The old emotions keep on recreating and recurring, over and over again, sometimes for an entire lifetime.

If we use memory reconsolidation in a conscious way, we can gain a sense of calm regarding these old memories. Amazingly, this transformation to calm can happen, quickly, easily, and permanently. You are not building new habits with this process. You are literally replacing emotional peptides, and the replacement process is simply to activate the old and replace with the new.

Let me now show you the three steps of using memory reconsolidation in a conscious and deliberate way. I use the acronym ICE, which stands for

Identify, Calm, Exchange

Identify:

When you activate a memory, you feel the old emotional peptide. Allow yourself to feel and identify this emotion. Most upsetting emotions can be identified as an anger, fear, or sadness.

In the automatic mode, you would recreate more of these same peptides and your memory would reglue back together with the same anger, fear, or sadness emotion. In conscious memory reconsolidation mode, you enter the calm state to deliberately create a different emotional state.

Calm:

When you observe two points and then space with nothing in it, you create a different emotional state and you also create a peptide corresponding to that new emotion of calm. This becomes the new instruction for your body. If you create calm, you will notice that your body returns to a relaxed state. The important part of the calm peptide is that it now becomes the glue available for regluing the synapses together in the old activated memory.

Exchange:

The last step in memory reconsolidation is to replace the old peptide with the new calm peptide. Look back and pay attention again to the original memory and the original emotion, exactly as they first occurred to you. Once you have created a calm peptide or some other alternative emotional peptide, this conscious observation of the old state allows the new calm peptide to reglue the old memory. Old troubled emotional peptides are replaced with calm.

The ICE Method is a practical application of the science of memory reconsolidation. Researchers first observed the effect in mice. By injecting certain chemicals into mouse brains they could remove the fear that had been trained into the mice. The first discoveries were made in the New York laboratory of Professor Joseph LeDoux, by Karim Nader and Glenn Schafe. In 2010, Nature Magazine published the first results of a study of human beings who eliminated a shock-induced fear response. Lead author Daniella Schiller titled the article, *Preventing the return of fear in humans using reconsolidcation uptake mechanisms.*[11] Testing participants a full year after the experiment showed that memory reconsolidation effects endured.

What difference does this discovery make? If therapy processes don't recognize how old emotions can truly replace with calm, then the best those therapies can offer is a "counteractive" approach, or "habit adaptation,"

Counteractive therapies help clients gain awareness of critical issues and then work to create alternative habits. Counteractive therapies help the client develop a different reaction to the terrors and debilitating effects of the past. Critically, though, since no memory reconsolidation replacement took place, the original emotion remains stored in the synapses of the old memories. When we create new habits, we are still reacting to old peptides. Habits give us a way to work around stored peptides, but the old peptides remain.

In terms of health those old emotions that remain stuck in our bodies can continue to push us towards fight-or-flight responses, creating a level of constant stress. Because most of us still believe in the permanence of our emotional history, the counteractive approach continues to dominate the solutions offered by pastors, therapists, counselors, rehabilitation workers, and self-help practitioners. Habit manipulation remains our primary tool. Unfortunately, changing habits doesn't change the underlying stored emotional peptides, and the underlying stresses remain as well.

Memory reconsolidation offers the promise that calm peptides can replace the emotions of even our most terrible memories and traumas. Instead of always reacting to old memories, we can replace peptides and create calm. When this happens we can experience freedom to create new possibilities without remaining stuck in our old emotions. The old emotions are replaced with the molecules of calm.

A personal note; my journey into healing has been shaped by EFT, the Emotional Freedom Technique introduced by Gary Craig in 1994. The process uses tapping on acupuncture points and directly addressing negative emotions in a person's life. EFT worked so well that I became captivated by the question of what actually happens to help people experience such huge physical and emotional changes.

In a multi-year reading quest I finally came upon the scientific phenomenon of memory reconsolidation.

My first exposure was a single paragraph in Joseph LeDoux's book, *The Synaptic Self*, published in 2002.[12] Pursuing that first tip, I eventually came to believe that when a person experiences emotional healing and related physical healing, regardless of the process or the therapy used, the process of memory reconsolidation has been involved.

With this conviction I started looking at EFT and other methods of healing for signs of memory reconsolidation in action. From that investigation I started modifying my EFT approach to take advantage of memory reconsolidation as directly as possible. This is The ICE Method I am sharing with you in this book – three simple steps.

Step 1 – I: Identify the non-calm issue

Step 2 – C: Calm your state of being

Step 3 – E: Exchange peptides

These three simple steps define The ICE Method and it can serve you for the rest of your life. For any non-calm situation that is not an actual physical threat you can use The ICE Method on the emotion and return your body and your mind to a state of calm.

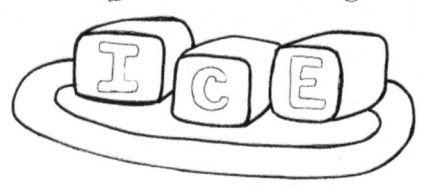

Identify. Calm. Exchange.

5 – ICE Your Past

In this chapter I will show you how to reconsolidate your old memories. The ICE Method works by bringing calm emotions to old traumas. When we look at the typical high-stress history of a person with fibromyalgia, the benefit of calming emotions becomes obvious.

Many people with fibromyalgia can identify one or more situations of trauma in their early life. The trauma does not have to include sexual abuse, but people with fibromyalgia do commonly report some kind of trauma or abuse. Because of the early trauma that people with fibromyalgia typically grew up with, the body forms the habit of constant preparation for danger. As a result, many people with fibromyalgia have grown up with their fight-or-flight stress response stuck in the ON position. The early trauma has caused lifelong stress on the body. Imagine setting the parking brake on your car and driving with the brake always on. Just as the car will damage more quickly, so too a body in constant stress mode will develop more symptoms. (Thank you to Dr. Ginevra Liptan for her book, *Figuring Out Fibromyalgia*, an important resource for understanding fibromyalgia and how it is impacted by the fight-or-flight response.)[13]

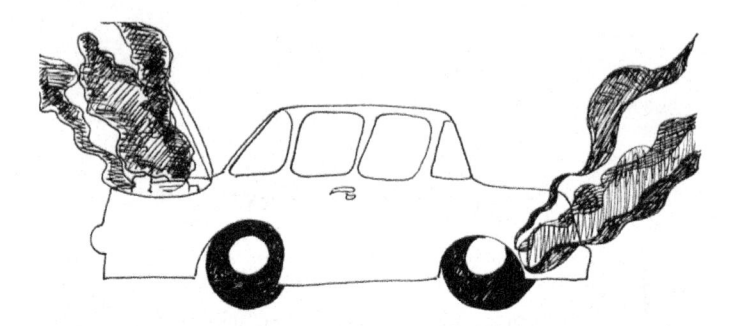

Sometime later in life, typically in their twenties or thirties, a person begins to feel the symptoms of fibromyalgia. Many people can remember a stressful triggering event that resulted in pain. The pain started at the time of that experience and then never went away. The triggering event could have been anything stressful from a car accident to a divorce, from a family emergency to physical or emotional abuse. In terms of stress, the triggering event looks like the straw that broke the camel's back; years or decades of stress wearing the body down to such a level it can finally no longer maintain function. One big event breaks the camel's back and the cascade of symptoms begins.

Why does the calming of emotions matter so much? When you use memory reconsolidation to clear the emotional pressure of old traumas, then your fight-or-flight stress response turns off. When the stress response stops then the body calms and turns to rest, restoration, and healing. Turning off your past stress history opens the door to healing. When you're in the calm state your body will do what it's meant to do – cells will focus on healing rather than protection, and restoration rather than defense. Whatever your body is capable of doing to improve your health, it will do this when it's in the calm state. The ICE Method helps you return to this default health state of your body.

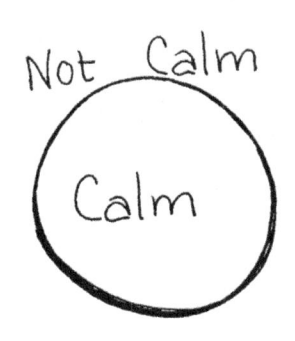

When you reconsolidate old memories, you grow your circle of calm. Observe that inside the calm space you feel calm. Outside the calm space you sense the stresses and anxieties of your life. So if you imagine the calm space as a circle, then there must be a boundary, an intersection between the calm space and the not-calm parts of your life.

Consider how great it would be if your calm space could be bigger? What if instead of having calm be some kind of special experience you could be calm most of the time? What if you could have calm be your default state? Here's how to create this for your life.

Step One – Identify

Begin by allowing the calm state to open up for you again. Use the two-point method and become aware of the space that has nothing in it. As a reminder, recall that you begin by observing a single point. Your body follows your mind as you do this simple thing.

Then observe a second point in the same manner. After doing this shift your attention to observing the space between the two points that has nothing in it. When you observe the space of nothing with your mind, you create calm peptides. These signal your body that there is nothing in the external world that requires a fight-or-flight response. The cells of your body go into rest and restoration mode. The chemistry of calm also now becomes available for memory reconsolidation. This space always resides with us, but we have so many other things going on we lose our awareness of this calm state. Let your awareness open up again.

We're going to focus on this boundary, the intersection between calm and not calm. Starting from the calm space, allow your focus to go out to the edge of the calm space. Notice the first thing that doesn't feel calm. You can have a specific memory in your mind before you begin, and if so, you can address this. Or you can simply go into the calm space and then take whatever you become aware of that does not feel calm.

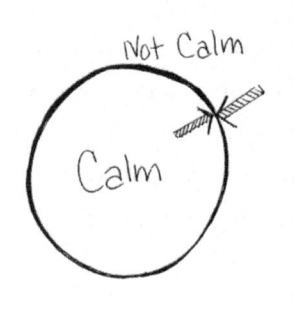

What comes up could be a memory, or an emotion you sense, or even a physical sensation in your body, something like nausea in the stomach, a constriction in the chest, tight back, pain in a joint or muscles, or headache. Look for any of the following three things:

- A physical sensation
- A specific memory
- An emotional feeling

Whatever you notice has likely stored in your body because of peptides. Peptides store our emotions. Peptides glue our memories. And peptides provide instructions to our bodies. This is why memories of a long ago trauma can make your body react right now. Using The ICE Method on whatever arises will stop this piece of your past from stressing your present. Whenever you use The ICE Method in this manner the reduction in stress load results in less pressure on your fibromyalgia symptoms.

Step Two – Calm

Whatever you noticed in Step One, physical, emotional, or a memory, these peptides have now activated. We can use the same reconsolidation process we used in Chapter Two for calming your emotion about having fibromyalgia.

We return from whatever agitation we observed outside of the calm circle and bring our attention back to our awareness of the calm state. Observe the two points again and the space in between. Spend a moment back in this peaceful state. Let your body enjoy being in its natural default state, focusing only on internal rest and restoration. Let your calm peptide bucket fill up and overflow so you can use your calm peptides to reconsolidate what you identified that was not calm.

Step Three - Exchange:

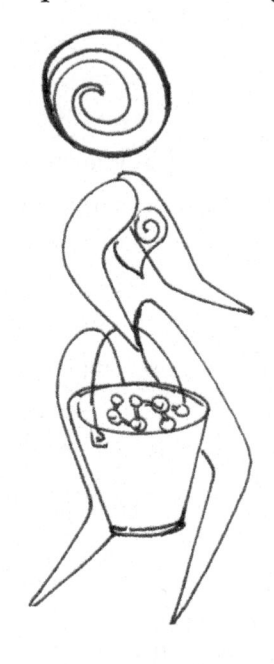

After a few moments in the calm state, focus again on whatever did not feel calm before, whether memory, emotion, physical sensation or some combination of those. Bring your bucket of calm peptides to observe again whatever did not feel calm. Because of the memory reconsolidation process, the activated peptides will be replaced with calm peptides. This will happen in your brain synapses, and it will also happen in your body where you felt sensations related to your memories or emotions. (Thanks to Candace Pert's, *Molecules of Emotions* for her work showing the link between peptides and body function. The fact that peptides also apply to storing body memories gives a powerful understanding for bringing calm and health to body and mind.)[14]

This is the ICE Method of memory reconsolidation. When you finish a round of observation, just notice what you notice. You do not need to hurry this process. Observe whatever shows up. If you really do go back and forth between the state of producing calm peptides and the state that did not feel calm, then reconsolidation will happen. What you observe as a result may or may not feel calm in a single go-round, but it will almost certainly feel different each time. Even if the same emotion still feels present, usually an aspect of the memory will have changed, or the sensation will appear in some other part of the body.

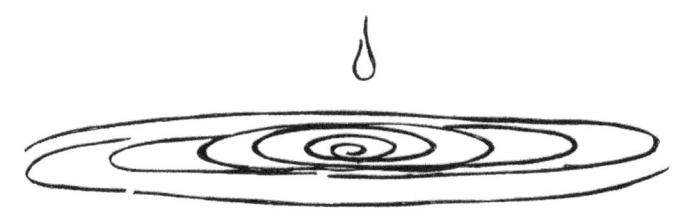

When I use the ICE Method, I imagine waves on a beach, back and forth between the calm and the not calm states, noticing what shows up as not calm and then repeating the process so I can observe it with calm peptides.

After working with many people for a wide variety of issues, I completely trust this process. One time I was working online via Skype with a fireman who said he had traumatic memories from his work arise as soon as he started the two point calming process. He had wanted to see me about his polymyalgia rheumatica, but his real issue was the anxiety and depression he was taking medication for.

"That's OK," I told him, "memory reconsolidation works by exchanging peptides between two different emotional states. Even if you're not calm, you are changing your emotional state just by paying conscious attention to the two points."

I did not feel confident after our first session, but a week later we were back for a second meeting and this man said he was using ICE all the time.

"I even went on an emergency call last week without any anxiety – it was like I was my old self back when I first started out as a firefighter."

I asked him about his polymyalgia rheumatica pain that he had first called me for. "It's gone," he said. During the second session we used The ICE Method again. A big memory came up during the session – getting benched as a kid during a baseball game. That had set the stage for a life of anxiety and perfectionism so that he'd never get caught getting benched again. Unfortunately, the high stress caused by living "on guard," all the time had ended up in disease. When we first met, he'd told me he thought his stress was eventually going to kill him. Using ICE, he went from distress about the baseball memory to only a few moments later finding himself chuckling about the incident. Memory reconsolidation allowed him to bring permanent calm to a memory that had compelled him to be on guard for many decades.

Four months after our first meeting, we visited by phone. I asked him about his polymyalgia rheumatica.

"It's still gone," he told me. "But I do have something I can't ICE on my own."

He went on to tell me he'd once suffered a severe panic attack at a breakfast restaurant. Ever since then he felt like vomiting if he went out for breakfast.

"I've been trying to ICE that but I just can't get to a calm space with it." We spent fifteen minutes on the phone together, just paying attention to whatever came up. By the end of our little mini-session he was looking forward to taking his wife out to breakfast again. You can always ICE on your own, but sometime an outside person can help identify stubborn issues and emotions.

Memory reconsolidation happens. It's a scientific and repeatable phenomenon. Applying the process may take a bit of practice and experience, but the science of reconsolidating emotional peptides in brain synapses is dependable. Back and forth. With this conscious process of Identifying, Calming, and Exchanging, you can enjoy the benefits of improved mind and body health.

The 3 steps of The ICE Method

1. **Identify:** Observe what does not feel calm.
2. **Calm:** Return to the calm state by observing two points and then observing the empty space in between them. Your body will follow your mind and your fight-or-flight response will turn off.
3. **Exchange**: Observe what did not feel calm and see what's different.

Continue this process and each time you make a loop, you will add more calm to the history of your life. Each time you bring more calm to the history of your life, you bring more calm to your present situation.

If you start using The ICE Method and begin to recognize its truly life-changing potential, you will want to keep coming back to this process and make it a part of your daily life. Whenever you notice you no longer feel calm, first check to see if you are facing any real immediate physical danger. If not, you can use The ICE Method and quickly return to the calm space. Then you can simply go back and forth with The ICE Method to reconsolidate whatever emotions, memories or physical sensations do not feel calm.

In the beginning, as you start making The ICE Method a part of your life, you might want to set a reminder alarm on your phone or watch. At first, set it to go off every five or so minutes and when the alarm rings, check to see if you're in the calm space. If not, find your two points and let the calm space open up for you again. The more you practice the more you'll discover that you're automatically staying in the calm space. At some point, after a few weeks or a month., you will likely discover that the calm state has become your normal state. Once calm becomes automatic, you'll immediately notice as soon as a non-calm emotion intrudes. Once calm has become your default state, it will be natural to use The ICE Method to reconsolidate the intruding emotion and then return to calm.

6 - Your Peptide Timeline

When we recall a memory, we react to the peptides stored in the synapses. Reacting to stress memories from the past can be a major cause of your fibromyalgia symptoms. In this chapter we will look at calming your peptide history as a way of reducing your fibromyalgia symptoms.

As best as I can understand, we used an emotional peptide to glue every memory we ever stored. If we didn't glue the memory with an emotional peptide, we wouldn't have a memory of that event. That's the nature of creating memories. We have literally stored a historical peptide timeline of everything that ever happened to us, an emotional history of all the times and all the places of your life. Everything we ever experienced and remembered – little peptide blips all along the historical timeline of your life.

Unless we reconsolidate the emotions we have of our past memories, we will continue reacting to the old emotion of each memory. Pleasant birthday party memories don't drain our energy, but past traumas can keep bringing old stress into our present life.

If we don't reconsolidate these memories with The ICE Method or some other process, then we can only continue living in reaction to our history. When a memory activates, we sense the emotion from the peptide which glued that memory together. When we feel the emotion, we react. If the emotion feels happy we gravitate toward similar actions. If the emotion feels fearful or angry, that emotion pushes us to fight or to flee from those situations. Unless we reconsolidate that old memory, the same response will surface every time the memory arises.

Take a kid who was bullied at school; she or he might have developed a real fear of being in public when they became adults. If that person doesn't reconsolidate the emotions about the bullying, he or she might end up using some traditional form of counteractive therapy. Such a process would try to help the person reach a new understanding of their childhood bullying memories. The process would continue by creating new habits so the person could hopefully learn to participate in public. The person would train themselves until they could better venture into public.

Counteractive processes use the brain's ability to create new brain cell wiring. This is called neuroplasticity. In effect, a new habit builds a new road in the brain so you can navigate around the old trauma memory. Building new habits is a major emphasis for helping people cope with early trauma. It takes a lot of work, and it often produces useful results. But new habits don't clear out the old emotional peptide. (In *Unlocking The Emotional Brain*, psychologist Bruce Ecker makes the case for how prevalently counteractive therapy is currently used, and how different the memory reconsolidation process is from the traditional counteractive therapies.)[15]

Counteractive therapy, building new habits to get around old traumas, has one major problem:

new habits do not remove old stored traumatic peptides.

Those old peptides remain stored in the synapses of the original trauma memories. For this reason habits require energy to maintain. Even a deeply learned habit still uses energy, because the old stored peptide remains. (For a clear explanation on brain function and habit-building, try Joe Dispenza's 2007 book, *Evolve Your Brain: The Science of Changing Your Mind*.)[16]

Habit building offers a powerful tool in almost everyone's life. Imagine, though, how much greater the power would be if we start out building our habits from a place of calm, instead of in reaction to stored peptides. If we use The ICE Method then we can replace our old trauma emotions with calm peptides. We can then create habits freely, beginning from a place of calm rather than from a place of emotional reactivity.

Using The ICE Method will make constructive habit building quicker. Using fibromyalgia as an example, imagine creating new habits as a way of coping with your pain. If the new habits still react to old emotions, then your fight-or-flight response is still turned on, still creating a stress within your body that can cause symptoms. Alternatively, if you use ICE, you will turn off your fight-or-flight stress response first. Then you will be free to create whatever habits you want, and your stress response will remain off.

Turn off the fight-or-flight response first; it will make a huge difference in your life.

Sometimes I imagine our lives resemble a pinball game. Pinball is like life without memory reconsolidation. When you play pinball, you launch a shiny metal ball onto a board filled with obstacles and rewards. Think of this board as your life, the obstacles and rewards correspond to your emotional peptide historical timeline. On this board you have flippers to keep the ball in play. You use the flippers to hit the rewards and avoid the obstacles. Yet, no matter the skill level of the player, without reconsolidation everyone does the same thing; react to existing obstacles and rewards.

If you add memory reconsolidation to the pinball game, you get a tool that lets you actually remove obstacles from the game, instead of just trying to avoid them. The obstacles and rewards represent the stored emotional peptides in your life. As you use The ICE Method, you remove stored peptides from the game of your life. Once removed, you can shoot the ball without interference. When you have cleared the old obstacles, then you can also freely create new memories and new habits to play a new game.

Without memory reconsolidation you're stuck playing the same pinball game for the rest of your life. This, I believe, consumes most of the lives of most of the people on our planet today. Let me say this again.

Most of us on this planet are living our lives as a *reaction* to the emotional peptides that have stored in our synapses.

These stored peptides from our past restrict our sense of what feels safe, and what feels good, and what seems dangerous. Look at how some people think its fine to speak in front of a packed auditorium and others would feel absolute terror in that situation. Why? Because each of them reacts to different stored peptides about what feels safe and what feels dangerous.

If we have a lot of energy, we develop great skill at reacting and navigating through the obstacles of the old pinball game of life. No matter how much energy and skill we have, though, we remain in reaction mode. Alternatively, if we have low energy, we may end up with a certain level of despair or depression. We may have little energy for playing the flippers to keep the ball moving. No matter one's energy or skill, though, without memory reconsolidation we will live life as a reaction to the emotional peptide history of our life.

Fibromyalgia Relief

The ICE Method gives us freedom to create a game of our own, making free choices rather than living in reaction to our past history.

The picture of a historical peptide timeline can help you in your healing. You now know that memory reconsolidation allows the possibility of replacing agitated peptides with calm ones. And you know The ICE Method provides you a process for accomplishing this. The image of a historical peptide timeline may be helpful for envisioning your history. Each time you use The ICE Method you make a specific piece of your history more calm.

Like the obstacles in any pinball game, each life has only a finite number of obstacles and rewards. Your emotional history is not an endless black hole you need to stay stuck in for the rest of your life. Using The ICE Method, you can address the pieces of your timeline one by one and achieve greater calm and peace in our life.

Does this still feel like too much work? Perhaps that's because you find yourself looking at this project from a state of agitation. If we're outside the circle of calm, we usually feel we must respond to stress with more stress. Try this.

Observe two points and then the empty space between them to open up a space of calm. From inside the circle of calm, consider and then answer the following question:

**Would I prefer to live my life
from a place of calm,
or from a place of stress and anxiety?**

If calm feels better, then choose calm. When something shows up that does not feel calm, no problem. Whenever non-calm shows up, as soon as you become aware of it, use The ICE Method on that peptide and return to calm. Simply do this as needed – your life will transform.

In this first part of *Fibromyalgia Relief*, you have discovered what I hope will be a life-changing process for improving your health and well-being. The science of how The ICE Method works will hopefully help the process make more sense to you. In this next part of *Fibromyalgia Relief* I want to look at what it might take for The ICE Method to become a part of your life. Transitioning from disease to health sounds like a goal we all want, but changes in health usually mean a change in our life patterns. Because we've been living in reaction to our stored peptides for all of our lives, we often can't believe or imagine a life beyond these constraints. In fact, many people react with fear when they first become aware that their life patterns really can change.

Unless we pay attention, we tend to revert to the old familiar, even when we know we want something new and better. To provide you with some more perspective, I next want to show you some examples of memory reconsolidation in everyday life. And then, to help you understand how the ICE Method complements and yet differs from traditional medical practice I want to share some insights and viewpoints from current medical practice and research.

PART TWO:

Stress

7 - How Long Will It Take?

I am often asked, "How long will it take for me to get better?

When we are ready, healing will take almost no time. Until we are ready, no time is enough. The process of memory reconsolidation has good scientific support, but we must feel a readiness to show up for healing before healing can begin. Engaging a healing process can feel threatening. In fact, a life of non-reactive freedom feels very different from living the old patterns of our history. Acting out of reaction to our history happens so regularly that even if we don't like the situation, we often take comfort in it's familiarity. When we feel ready to explore the journey forward from the old familiar to the new freedom, then symptom relief becomes far more possible.

I never guarantee how a person will feel physically after using The ICE Method. A person's pain situation may include more than reacting only to stored peptides. Yet neither do I discount what might be possible from using The ICE Method. I have worked with at least a dozen people who have experienced complete back pain relief even though their MRI photos show real physical damage including stenosis, misalignment, bulging discs, and even bone-on-bone contact because discs have worn away.

Depending on causes, healing experiences may vary. I do not know what results a person will achieve, but I do have great confidence in the improvements that arise when we address and replace agitated peptides with calm peptides. The feeling of calm puts us in a health-creating state, both emotionally and physically. If you're motivated to have good health, no matter what else you do, this calm space is the place from which to live your life.

The list of stress-related and immune-response related issues and diseases includes a huge range that extends from fibromyalgia to some cancers, and from diabetes and Parkinson's to some back pains and to some heart diseases. No matter what ails a person, The ICE Method offers benefits just by calming a person's peptides and letting the cells of their body operate in rest and restoration mode.

Are you ready to live from this calm place?

Since most of us have spent our lives reacting to our stored peptides without any knowledge that we could change them, it becomes a real question, whether we actually feel prepared to start living from a calm state. Those stored peptides of the past have provided us with an unconscious system, a roadmap for automatically assessing what feels safe and what feels dangerous. Why do some professionals race NASCAR for a living while others feel tense in regular freeway traffic? Answer - stored peptides from experiences long ago.

Peptides have stored in reaction to every situation we have experienced in life. Ever since those experiences we have reacted to the stored peptides as a guide to our present choices. The problem is this: peptides stored from a childhood incident decades ago do not necessarily provide the best information for how to react to all current situations. Think about this for a moment and you can see how a life of reactive decision making can cause so much stress on our mind and body.

I did a study where I discovered just how much our stored peptides and reactivity can shape our healing. In the fall of 2012 I spent time at a fibromyalgia clinic, offering a single ICE Method session to each of 39 people with fibromyalgia.

For the first 13 people I used what turned out to be a less-effective method for helping people become aware of the calm state. It gave an interesting result. For the seven who felt the experience of the calm state, all of them experienced complete elimination of their pain during the session. The six who did not enter a calm state experienced little or no pain relief. Calm matters.

When I modified the approach and started using the two-point calm-space technique of this book, then the results became even better. Every one of the remaining 26 patients in the study entered the calm state. Of these, twenty-one experienced complete pain relief during their session. The remaining five all experienced significant relief, but not the complete elimination of their pain during the single session. All these patients were under care at a clinic specializing in fibromyalgia care. Most of these patients had severe symptoms as assessed by their caregiver and as reported on the FIQR (Revised Fibromyalgia Impact Questionnaire.). FIQR scores ranged from 30 to 91 with an average of 62.

For the 33 patients who did enter the calm space, the following graph shows their self-reported pain levels prior to their single session.

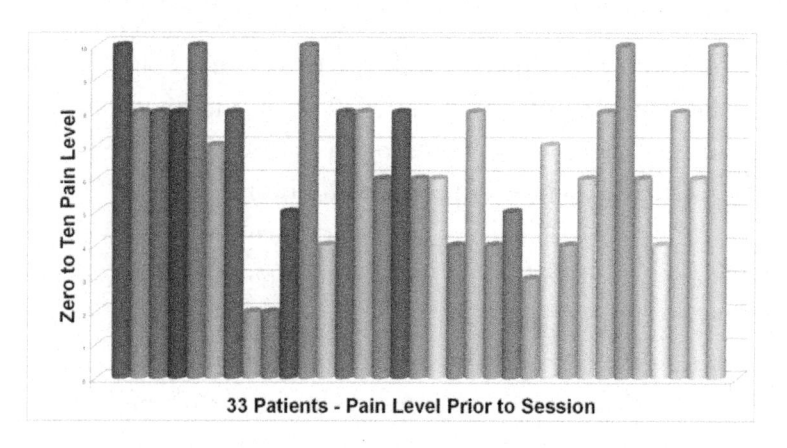

33 Patients - Pain Level Prior to Session

The next graph shows the self-reported pain levels for each of these patients after a single ICE Method session. This study is part of what inspired me to write *Fibromyalgia Relief*. But it also raised a new question.

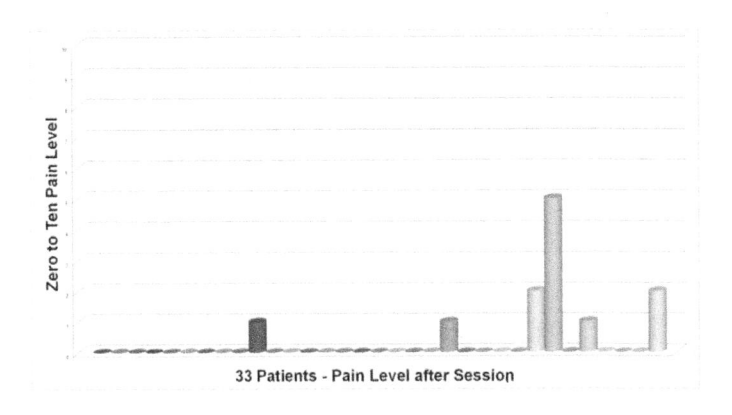

33 Patients - Pain Level after Session

I expected that all of these people who experienced pain relief would enjoy lasting results. Their experience of the calm state allowed their fight-or-flight response to shut off and the resulting rest state for their body allowed their pain to abate. At worst, I expected that if pain returned they would accept my invitation to call me again for another session. I had given contact information to each person. I had even called and emailed everyone for follow-up. Of all these people, only one phoned me back. Only a few returned my emails. The rest did not reply. Their health-care provider reported to me that pain levels had returned again by their next patient visits.

It appears that if you've suffered pain for a long time, then becoming pain free necessitates a psychic change in your life – a change in spirit. Looking back, I realize I had surprised these patients by showing up at their regular medical appointments. They had not come to their appointment that day prepared for a medical possibility of having zero pain. They had come for a regular appointment and then their medical care provider had explained what I do and invited them to experience a session right after their regular appointment. So the pain elimination came as an unexpected surprise.

Eliminating a person's pain may also have caused an upset to the coping routines these patients had established over many years. Some of these patients had so much pain they qualified for disability status. Some had undergone back surgeries and other major procedures to treat their pain. Each of these patients had relationships that would change if they became fully functional again. All of these patients had a long personal history with pain. For any of us, when we experience big changes in our life, we have to put the pieces together again in a new way.

One of the patients later told his doctor that the experience with me had been "weird and not useful." This patient had arrived at his appointment with level ten pain in his joints. I remember him saying, "If you could cut these legs off right now to get rid of the pain, go ahead and take them." Within fifteen minutes of being introduced to The ICE Method, his pain had disappeared completely. For the first time in years, he walked out of the fibromyalgia clinic pain free.

Yet, although this man experienced complete pain relief in his physical body, his mind interpreted the experience as, "weird and not useful." I did have one brief phone conversation with this patient a week after this session. It was only a minute long–he answered his phone while rushing to a store to get ready for a trip. He didn't have time to talk to me. He was back in stress mode. His fight-or-flight response was turned on again. Calm seemed like a "weird and not useful" tool to bring to the stress of his life. The pain had returned full force.

When we are in fight-or-flight mode, calm may not feel like a solution, calm may even feel dangerous.

Witnessing pain disappear for these patients served as a real confirmation of the usefulness of The ICE Method. My experience is that if The ICE Method can bring pain relief in one session, then it will be useful again should pain return; it usually just means there's another emotional trigger to be addressed.

The "weird and not useful" feedback, though, is what turned out to be the most valuable for me. From experiences like this I came to understand that lasting pain relief often involves far more than simply eliminating the sensation of pain. I took one major question away from this study: "How do we best help people make their healing *last*?"

For healing to endure, I have come to believe that three things can help produce better results when working with the ICE method.

Readiness:

A readiness to step into the changes that will come with healing. This readiness sets the pace at which healing can proceed. Each of us chooses a pace that makes sense to our life experience. Since old emotional peptides dominate our lives until we use The ICE Method (or some other similarly effective process), a reactive fear of change can impede our ability to embrace the healing process.

Science:

An understanding of the science of The ICE Method can increase our openness to healing. Once a person understands the memory reconsolidation mechanism, healing our peptide history becomes a predictable process. A willingness to make The ICE Method an ongoing part of our life becomes easier as we experience an expanding circle of calm. Healing experiences move from the realm of magic to a scientifically predictable process of putting our body into its natural calm and healing state.

Spirit

I have also come to believe that the personal stresses we bear are part of living in a culture and a world that carries an enormous accumulation of collective stress. The isolating worldview of "survival of the fittest" leaves us with constant background fear and a fight-or-flight response that can easily end up stuck in the ON position. We benefit when we understand ourselves as part of some greater whole.

Living from the calm space can grow our sense of connection to others, to our world, and even to the world of spirit. Healing our physical bodies involves more than just how well our body parts function. In Part Three I will open up some thoughts about anthropology, spiritual traditions, and quantum science.

The history of our mechanical, individual separateness has only come to dominate our global outlook in the past hundreds of years. The decrease in social connection and the increase in material attachment seems to me a major factor in the rise of fight-or-flight malfunctions and immune system disorders. For healing to last, I believe we benefit by including our spirit, as well as our body and our mind.

As I've said now many times in this book, make the calm state your default state. When you live in the calm state, you will automatically start dissolving whatever fears or worries hold you back from engaging in healing. The calm state brings peace.

In the next chapter you'll read of four situations where memory reconsolidation happens naturally, without a person even being aware of the peptide chemistry involved. Before sharing these examples, I want to reflect on healing for just a bit.

Sometimes we interpret our experience as a healing. Other times we do not. How do we define healing? How do we talk about healing?

I worked once with a man for his back pain. He was on legal disability status. When his thirty years of back pain disappeared he felt an initial sense of wonderment and joy, which turned quickly to worry. "How can I tell my friends all this pain disappeared just by looking at nothing?"

Healing literally means, "to make whole." And then, like this man, when it happens we try our best to explain what we experienced. Out of this process and through the ages have arisen countless healing modalities, countless explanations for the process and the experience of healing. Ten years ago I would never have predicted I would be part of exploring, experiencing, and explaining the process of physical healing. I write these words now because my wish is for you to have your own experience of healing from the symptoms of fibromyalgia. If you find a way forward through these words – fantastic. If you find help through other means – equally excellent.

For the remainder of this book I'm going to push on from the technique of The ICE Method and the science of memory reconsolidation. I invite you into my own personal conversation about what makes healing happen, and the underlying causes we need to heal from. If my journey adds something to your journey, great. If not, I trust you'll find the connections through other words for healing, health, and living in our modern world.

How we understand the world makes a difference to our symptoms of fibromyalgia. If we suffer because our fight-or-flight response is stuck in the ON position, this involves both our personal health and also our relationship with our environment, our context, and the world we live in. You can stick with the first part of this book and likely feel better just by using The ICE Method presented in these first chapters. Or you can read on as I explore what might be a more complete answer for why you healed than just telling your friends, "I learned to observe a space with nothing in it!"

As you explore healing further, through this book and other resources, I hope you will find health and wholeness making more sense and hopefully being more present in your life of body, mind, and spirit.

8 – It's Everywhere

Memory reconsolidation exists everywhere. Let's look at how it shows up in everyday life. Since the laboratory discovery dates back only to 2004, very few people have the scientific understanding for recognizing memory reconsolidation in action. Of course, even without people being aware of the brain chemistry, memory reconsolidation happened in brain synapses every time memories were activated. To help you get a better feel for the memory reconsolidation process, here are four examples from priests, grandmothers, best friends, and practitioners of the Emotional Freedom Technique (EFT).

I hope that by reading these examples you will begin recognizing memory reconsolidation happening in your daily life. Before the examples, let me recommend two resources for more on memory reconsolidation. First, you may want to search the Internet for references and for scholarly papers about memory reconsolidation. New publications appear as the research continues. Also, as I mentioned, a major article was published in Nature Magazine in 2010,

"Preventing the return of fear in humans using reconsolidation update mechanisms."[17] Second, you may want to read the first full book published about using memory reconsolidation. I've mentioned this book already, written by psychiatrists Bruce Ecker, Robin Ticic, and Laurel Hully.[18] *Unlocking The Emotional Brain* shares the process that these and other psychiatrists have developed for using memory reconsolidation in their therapy sessions. Their method has more technicalities than The ICE Method and requires trained therapists to use the method. Their technique is proving to be very effective with their clients. I believe that *Unlocking the Emotional Brain* is an early example of how memory reconsolidation will ultimately evolve into our general awareness and everyday use. Now on to the examples.

Catholic confession provides an example of memory reconsolidation in action. You rob a bank and you feel terrible. You worry about capture and feel the emotion of fear. As you tell the priest about the robbery, the stored peptides of fear activate. The priest listens. Here in the confessional your environment has changed. Worn oak panels surround you inside the booth, footsteps echo gently on the stone floor outside. Light filters in through stained glass. Your state of emotion changes as the priest listens in silence. You enter a calm state. After the story, the priest speaks the words of forgiveness. Regardless of what happens in the celestial realms, when the state of calm is brought to the bank robber's state of fear, peptides exchange in a process of memory reconsolidation. Calm peptides replace the fear peptides of the bank robbery.

As with confessing to a priest, if you are a person who prays, you may sometimes notice that after you bring up an upsetting issue in prayer, as you begin to remember the goodness and the help of the One you pray to, a sense of peace replaces the agitation you felt about the issue. Along with whatever divine intervention you may be experiencing, this going back and forth between the agitation of your issue and the peace of your God can parallel the process of memory reconsolidation.

Grandmothers, too can also provide memory reconsolidation as powerful as priests. Imagine a bloody nose after a childhood fight with the boy down the street. Home you run with tears in your eyes and trembling anger in your body.

"Sit right here," Grandma says, helping you into a chair at the kitchen table. She gets a warm wet cloth for your beaten nose. The cookie jar comes off the shelf and two fresh-baked cookies appear on a napkin. In another moment a cup of hot cocoa also arrives.

"Now tell me all about it," Grandma says. Sugar replaces anger. Love blankets the fight of a few moments before. Memory reconsolidation transforms the emotion from anger to calm.

Your best friend tells you she'll be right over. Your tears keep falling into your pillow even when she arrives, the ending of the relationship as fresh as if the breaking-up words had not yet finished. Your friend holds you tight. No words pass. Sadness eventually replaces with calm. The chemistry of peptide exchange, memory reconsolidation, brings you back to life again. If your friend had not been available, you would likely have spent the whole night in your tears, and the emotions would have remained the same because no reconsolidation happened. Although we haven't had the scientific data for memory reconsolidation before, we've witnessed its effects through experiences such as confession with a priest, comfort from a grandmother, or the heart-to-heart listening of a best friend.

One last example I would like to share with you, this one from EFT, short for the Emotional Freedom Technique. It's popular, simple, and from my own experience highly effective. The technique uses tapping with your fingers against acupuncture points on your body. At the same time as you tap you speak words about whatever physical or emotional issue you are struggling with. You name whatever emotion you feel. Also, at the beginning of each session you do a step that I believe engages memory reconsolidation. Each session starts with words about the specific issue, such as a headache. "Even though I have this terrible tension headache right behind my eyes, I deeply love and accept myself."

The headache has one emotional state. "Love and acceptance" provides the alternate state. As you can see once again, memory reconsolidation happens when you activate a memory and then you move your observation back and forth between emotional states and calm.

Once you experience memory reconsolidation, and once you understand the mechanism, you begin to notice emotional peptides all around you. Sometimes reconsolidation changes the peptides, but in many cases you observe that people's emotions appear reactive and stuck. The personal grudges; the hardened political stances; the automatic assumptions made about insiders and outsiders; these often seem frozen and unopen to peptide replacement. From an understanding of peptides it becomes clear how commonly people make the reactive choice instead of replacing emotional peptides and operating from calm freedom. As more and more people grow aware of the memory reconsolidation process, I believe we will start seeing its conscious use in new and exciting ways.

I'll mention one more time how highly I recommend you make the calm space your default state. Transforming your life from reactivity to calm freedom will change your life in ways impossible to imagine until the journey begins. And whatever difference you make for yourself, you also become the possibility of helping other people understand and work with their own historical peptide timeline.

In the next chapter I will share some information about research and medical perspective on fibromyalgia. The incidence of fibromyalgia and many other stress-related diseases continues to rise around the world.

Different doctors approach these diseases in different ways. It turns out the assumptions and beliefs one has about medicine make a big difference. Perhaps most importantly is whether we believe the function of the mind affects the function of the body. As you discovered for yourself in the earlier part of this book, your own view about fibromyalgia makes a pivotal difference in the level of pain you experience. Understanding that mind and body connect through emotions and through emotional peptides provides a new avenue for healing.

After we consider body, mind, and fibromyalgia in the next chapter, we'll move to Part Three where I invite you to join me and consider how our changing world may be creating the stress conditions for the increase of fibromyalgia and many other diseases.

9 – Body, Mind, and Fibromyalgia

The theory behind The ICE Method is that we produce molecules (peptides) that correspond to our emotional state. These molecules provide instructions to our cells. Using the ICE Method we shift our emotional state to calm so the cells of the body can enter a calm state of rest and restoration.

A young boy just starting high school came to see me recently. He was experiencing, "the most painful summer of my life." He'd been hospitalized twice for severe stomach and chest pains, and doctors were continuing to look for causes.

"I don't know what we can do about your pains," I told him, "I never know what the physical result will be, but I'm pretty sure we can get the cells of your body into a rest state so they can focus on whatever healing is possible for you."

Within a few moments he was laughing, "this feels good," he told me, "the 'nothing feeling' makes me laugh." After a few moments in the calm space I asked about the pain in his stomach and chest.

"It's gone, I feel fine now," he told me. On its own, the calm space often allows for remarkable health improvements, whether its fibromyalgia or other issues.

These peptide molecules also do a second function in The ICE Method; they replace the emotions of our stored memories using the process of memory reconsolidation.

For this boy with the stomach and chest issues, he told me about the stress he has around being a leader on his sports team. I asked him to let himself recall and feel the emotion of one of the stressful situations from the last year.

"Now do the calm space again," I invited him., after he had accessed the feeling of anger. Then after he was comfortably back to calm, "Now look back and observe that exact same situation again. Tell me if it feels the same or different."

"It feels different. It's like I'm just looking at those players, but I'm not angry at them anymore."

"That," I told him, is how you can calm any stressful memories from the past or worries about the future. If it's not going to cause you immediate physical harm, you don't need to carry any stress about it. If you decide to do this as part of your life, I think your chest and stomach are going to keep feeling better.

Up to this point we've been about peptides and synapses to get these kinds of results using The ICE Method. Now we're going to look at the specific relationship of emotions and peptides to fibromyalgia..

You've already learned the technique of The ICE Method, so if you find parts of this chapter too technical, just give it a quick skim for whatever you might find useful. Mostly what I want out of this chapter is for you to see that research exists to support the connection between fibromyalgia, emotions, stress and peptides.

As we've already discovered, peptide molecules, "the molecules of emotion," are a big deal. Whenever you use The ICE Method to calm past emotions, memory reconsolidation allows you to replace peptide molecules in your brain.

It turns out that peptide molecules also receive and send instructions in your immune system. And it's the job of the immune system to protect you from outside microbes and to provide healing after injuries and disease. Inside the brain there are other cells that function much like the white cells of the immune system outside. Inside the brain they get a different name, glial cells. These cells are one of the current research emphases related to fibromyalgia.[19][20][21] A properly functioning immune system can tell the difference between the self it is protecting and the invaders who are attacking. A malfunctioning immune system may start attacking the body it is supposed to protect.

What does this have to do with fibromyalgia? Peptides. Scientists used to believe that the immune system functioned automatically, independently of our conscious mind. Then in the early 1980's Candace Pert and Michael Ruff[22] discovered that each of the brain cell peptide receptors (the stuff we access when we use The ICE Method,) also exist on immune cell membranes. Since brain cell peptides form in response to emotions, it turns out that the immune system also responds to our conscious mind. Our emotions create peptides and peptides direct the activity of the white blood cells in our body and the glial cells in our brain and central nervous system. Physical body and conscious mind connect through our immune system. With a tool such as The ICE Method, we have the ability to consciously influence at least some of the immune functions that protect our body and brain.

Dr. Pert explains her growing awareness of this connection as she began a practice of meditation: (At the time of her writing the connection to glial cells in the brain had not yet been developed.)

> With my knowledge of the bodywide psychosomatic network, I was beginning to think of disease-related stress in terms of an information overload, a condition in which the mind-body network is so taxed by unprocessed sensory input in the form of suppressed trauma or undigested emotions that it has become bogged down and cannot flow freely, sometimes even working against itself at cross-purposes…When stress prevents the molecules of emotion from flowing freely where needed, the largely autonomic

processes that are regulated by peptide flow such as breathing, blood flow, immunity, digestion, and elimination collapse down to a few simple feedback loops and upset the normal healing response.[23]

In the Calm step of The ICE Method, the two-point process of becoming aware of the calm space has many similarities to meditation. Pert describes it this way: "Meditation, by allowing long-buried thoughts and feelings to surface, is a way of getting the peptides flowing again, returning the body and emotions to health."[24]

Research since about the year 2000 began to more deeply explore the role of micro-glia and astrocytes, the specialized cells that inhabit the brain and central nervous system. Linda Watkins begins an extensive review paper from 2007 with these words:

> It is recently become clear that activated immune cells and immune-like glial cells can dramatically alter neuronal function. By increasing neuronal excitability, these non-neuronal cells are now implicated in the creation and maintenance of pathological pain, such as occurs in response to peripheral nerve injury.[25]

In other words, when the immune system excites the nerves too much, it hurts. Watkins then goes on to give a description of neuropathic pain that will be familiar to many with fibromyalgia.

Neuropathic pain is a form of pathological pain that arises from trauma, inflammation and/or infection of peripheral nerves. Here, sensations from the affected body region are grossly abnormal. Environmental stimuli that would never normally be perceived as pain now are, and environmental stimuli that are normally perceived as painful now elicit amplified perceptions of pain. In addition, environmental stimuli may evoke abnormal perceptions of electric tingling or shocks (paraesthesias) and/or sensations having unusually unpleasant qualities (dysesthesias). Lastly, spontaneous pain frequently occurs with varying qualities and from varying perceived body locations.[26]

If the immune system starts attacking the cells of the body and results in physical damage to the body, this is labeled autoimmunity. Fibromyalgia is not listed as an autoimmune disease, because researchers have not identified actual tissue damage arising from this disease. Still, even though fibromyalgia is not autoimmune, immune peptides are involved in the experience of symptoms and pain. In 2008, Jay Shah and Elizabeth Gilliams published their study of the chemistry of myofascial trigger points. When they sampled trigger point fluid they found it contained all the markers of an immune system response. When the trigger points were relieved the immune system markers no longer remained.[27]

In 2012, a study led by Frederick Behm used a different method of testing for immune peptide response in people with fibromyalgia. He tested for eight different peptides and found significantly different levels for seven of them, concluding that "cell-mediated immunity is impaired in fibromyalgia patients.[28]

In a 2010 study led by R.J. Tynan, researchers focused on the effect of the chronic stress which is such a familiar part of people's experience of fibromyalgia. They found that "chronic stress selectively increases the number of microglia in certain stress-sensitive brain regions."[29]

Translation - more stress results in more pain.

In a 2009 study, Shuei Sugama also found that acute stress activates microglia and increases activity in an area of the brain that responds to uncontrollable stress, threat, anxiety and pain.[30]

This is a lot of medical information to absorb. If you're interested you can start with these studies and do as much of your own research as you wish. If you're not all that curious about the medical research being done, that's fine too, just know that many of the researchers are interested in peptides, and The ICE Method is all about peptides.

Not too long ago, many doctors dismissed fibromyalgia as nothing more than an "emotional" disease, that there was nothing really wrong with a person. Now, through the studies being done, I believe we are coming closer to understanding the connection between mind and body and the possibilities for honoring and improving our health.

One more area of study to mention – another possible cause of fibromyalgia pain is a condition called small fiber neuropathy, occurring from damage to the small peripheral nerve fibers. People with neuropathy can have reduced sensitivity in their feet, legs, hands, and arms. A 2013 study by N Uceyler and a team of researchers compared small fiber neuropathy in people with fibromyalgia to those who didn't have fibromyalgia. Ucelyr found fewer small fiber nerves in the body for people with fibromyalgia, possibly a cause for pain.[31] In a study by Anne Louise Oaklander she tested a group of people with fibromyalgia and found 50% of them tested positive for small fiber neuropathy.[32] In the control group of people who didn't have fibromyalgia, no one tested positive for small fiber neuropathy. In terms of possible connections to immune response, small fiber neuropathy is a common pain issue for many kinds of autoimmune disease such as diabetes, lupus, etc. Is there a connection to peptides and to the possibilities for health? To me it seems possible, and even likely.

Whether or not fibromyalgia someday makes the official list of autoimmune diseases, if the results of these studies hold, then immunological disorder, stress, and the fight-or-flight response provide an important avenue for understanding fibromyalgia and how The ICE Method works. Accessing the calm state can change our body peptides and this can change the response of our immune system.

Emotions and stress make up a big part of our environment We know that emotions cause the production of peptides, and peptides are involved in almost all parts of our life, including body function, brain activity, memory storage, and immune function.

Once you start observing the physical effects of emotional stress, and especially once you start experiencing the power of the Calm space to turn off the fight-or-flight stress response, you may join the growing numbers who are seeking out the connections between mind, body, and spirit. Even though change comes slowly, after hundreds of years of Descarte's mind/body split, we now live in a time where the medical and research fields are beginning to break down the separate treatment of mind and body.

One of these steps forward in recognizing the mind/body connection comes from Dr. Ginevra Liptan's *Figuring Out Fibromyalgia: Current Science and the Most Effective Treatments*. A fibromyalgia sufferer herself, a medical researcher, and a practicing physician, Liptan writes plainly,

> Ultimately all the symptoms of fibromyalgia stem from abnormal activation of the fight-or-flight nervous system.[33]

Liptan goes on to state her case even more strongly. (emphasis mine.)

The muscles and fascia of the body are clenched in fibromyalgia in constant preparation for fight or flight...Medical science has not yet figured out how to turn off the switch of the stress response that gets stuck in the ON position in fibromyalgia. *When we do that we will have found a cure.*[34]

I believe that The ICE Method, unlike Western medical science, actually does provide a way to turn off our fight/flight/freeze response. This shutting off of the stress response results in the relief of symptoms experienced by people with fibromyalgia. I have a feeling that big and positive changes lie ahead as traditional medicine begins to include mind/body connections more intentionally.

Another doctor who bridges mind and body served patients as a family doctor and palliative care specialist in Canada. Dr. Gabor Maté did something unusual for a practicing doctor; he interviewed his patients at length and spent extended time learning their life stories and patterns. In the process of comparing their stories he made a valuable discovery - similar life history patterns often resulted in similar diseases. Dr. Maté's interviews matched what he found in many scientific studies: specific life stressors often coincide with specific diseases.

Dr. Maté provides an well-documented thesis for his link between life stresses and particular diseases. While reading *When The Body Says NO*,[35] I realized that the usefulness of The ICE Method may extend to relieving some autoimmune diseases as well as fibromyalgia. I want to share with you how Dr. Maté describes autoimmunity and disease.

> In autoimmune disease, the body's defenses turn against the self...Within the physical organism, physical mutiny results from an immunological confusion that perfectly mirrors the unconscious psychological confusion of self and non-self."[36]

As I noted earlier, many people with fibromyalgia, and it turns out many people with autoimmune disease, have experienced early trauma and stress in their lives. Dr. Maté listened to hundreds of these stories as he interviewed his patients. Based on his interviews, he believed that these traumas led to a loss of personal psychological boundaries between the body and its physical environment. Their stressed environments became toxic to their health. Continuing with Dr. Maté,

> In this disarray of boundaries, the immune cells attack the body as if the latter were a foreign substance, just as the psychic self is attacked by inward-directed reproaches and anger...
>
> The cross confusion reflects disruptions of the interconnected body/mind mechanisms within the emotional-nervous-immune hormonal supersystem ... If immune cells that turn against the self are not destroyed or made harmless, they will attack the body tissues they were meant to guard. Allergic reactions or autoimmune diseases may result."[37]

Long term stress can result in immune malfunction. Understanding stress provides a basis for why The ICE Method works. In this chapter I hope you are gaining some confidence that medical evidence and medical studies point to how The ICE Method can promote the healing of fibromyalgia. From the medical voices of Dr. Pert, Dr. Maté, Dr. Liptan and others we can see the possibility of how long term stress and fight/flight/freeze activation have a part in what causes fibromyalgia symptoms.

We'll continue with Dr. Maté to see his explanation for how stress turns into disease.

> The stress response may be triggered in reaction to any attack – physical, biological, chemical, or psychological – or in response to any perception of attack or threat, conscious or unconscious. The essence of a threat is a destabilization of the body's homeostasis, the relatively narrow range of physiological conditions within which the organism can survive and function. To facilitate fight or escape, blood needs to be diverted from the internal organs to the muscles, and the heart needs to pump faster. The brain needs to focus on the threat, forgetting about hunger or sexual drive. Stored energy supplies need to be mobilized, in the form of sugar molecules. The immune cells must be activated. Adrenaline, cortisol and the stress substances fulfill those tasks."[38]

You see now why the calm state can feel so compelling and helpful? In the calm state you shut off your fight-or-flight stress response and your cortisol and adrenaline levels return from high alert back down to normal levels.

If you suffered an early trauma and your stress response got stuck in the ON position; no wonder your body eventually becomes exhausted and may even start experiencing disease such as fibromyalgia symptoms. As Dr. Maté describes,

> Chronically high cortisol levels destroy tissue. Chronically elevated adrenalin levels raise the blood pressure and damage the heart…There is extensive documentation of the inhibiting effect of chronic stress on the immune system.[39]

An astounding number of chemical reactions happen in your body when it responds to a stress event. If the body fails to return to calm and experiences long term conditions of chronic stress the immune system eventually breaks down and immune dysfunction begins. Studies show that the hippocampus in the brain literally shrinks in size and capacity because of too much cortisol. Memory impairment follows and the body's ability to regulate its own stress response also declines.[40] The amygdala becomes abnormally sensitized and more easily triggered at lower activation levels. The adrenal glands produce cortisol in response to chronic stress, but if the stress lasts long enough the body may lose its ability to produce enough cortisol. The natural anti-inflammatory action of cortisol no longer keeps inflammation in check. Inflammation can affect almost all the tissues of the body, including everything from cancer cell production to blood vessel inflammation to swelling joints and rheumatoid pain. Autoimmune diseases, fibromyalgia, and other conditions may result.

Traditional Western medicine has focused on treating the symptoms of fibromyalgia. As Dr. Liptan noted in her book, Western medicine treats symptoms because it hasn't figured out how to shut off the stress response. In her words, again, "when we figure out how to turn off the switch of the stress response that gets stuck in the ON position in fibromyalgia...we will have found a cure."[41]

Creating calm, as we've seen in the first part of this book, shuts off the fight-or-flight response. Creating calm, as Dr. Bruce Lipton has noted in *Biology of Belief*, puts cells in rest mode so they can attend to health, restoration, and healing. Creating calm, as Dr. Candace Pert has noted in *Molecules of Emotion*, changes the biochemistry of our brain and our body, including our immune system. As Pert discovered, even the immune system can create its own signaling peptides. Dr. Maté compared the immune system to a "floating brain in our bodies," carrying learned information about what is safe and what is dangerous for the survival of our body. Calm peptides allow our immune system to function freely rather than from a stress-induced reaction to perceptions of danger.

I hope this second part of *Fibromyalgia Relief* has provided you some background for understanding The ICE Method from both practical and medical perspectives. So far we have looked at the science of turning off our fight-or-flight stress response. We have learned a process for improving our physical and emotional health. Why, though, do we seem to have more stress now than in earlier times, both individually and in our society? And what can we do about this?

Part Three turns to consider possible causes and solutions to our modern day stress crisis from perspectives of history, anthropology, and spirituality.

PART THREE

Health in a Stress-filled World

10 – A Brief History of Stress

When I first got involved with healing, I focused on symptoms; the aching back, the sore arm, insomnia, tinnitus, neuropathy, the pains of fibromyalgia. When the symptoms disappeared I considered sessions successful. The study I made with the 39 fibromyalgia patients offered a wake-up call. Symptoms matter, but long-term physical healing involves more than symptom relief.

As you have discovered in learning and using The ICE Method, the key to relief of your fibromyalgia symptoms involves turning off your fight-or-flight stress response and keeping it turned off. As I discovered in my study with the fibromyalgia patients, turning off the fight-or-flight response happened predictably and provided dramatic relief. However, keeping that stress response turned off presents another level of engagement with your healing.

In Part One we learned about memory reconsolidation and how it can help us calm the emotions of our memories, even the emotions associated with trauma from early years. Consistently using the ICE Method on our current emotions and our past memories will help us shut down our fight-flight response and keep it turned off. If The ICE Method can provide such relief, why do some people discontinue using the process?

The simple answer to this question is that most of us have developed the habit of stressful situations being accompanied by a bodily stress-response. The stress response in our body doesn't actually help, because there's no physical action to be taken, yet this stress response of the body has become a habit whenever we face a stressful situation such as an overdue bill, a traffic jam, or a disagreement with our children.

The stress response feels familiar to us – even necessary.

If we ICE and choose calm instead of reactive stress, the feeling can be strange. Choosing Calm in the face of a perceived stress can even feel dangerous, as if we're not taking the threat seriously.

It's the rare moment when we face an actual physical threat to our immediate physical threat. Those uncommon moments are actually the only time we really need a fight-flight stress response to save us from harm. In all other circumstances, if we could learn to consistently shut off our fight/flight/freeze response, we'd be healthier.

In Part Three of this book, I invite you to join with me in considering the bigger picture of stress in our individual lives and the world we live in. Hopefully, this reflection about our life and our place in the world will make it easier for us to choose calm and make it our default state of being.

It may make more sense to choose calm if we spend some time reflecting on how our culture, religion, and science frame our worldviews and lead us to stress. Understanding how these affect our daily living may help us lower our stress. For this reason, I want to turn now toward a broader view of stress.

We'll look at how stress has grown in our culture - something like 75-90% of all visits to the doctor have their basis in stress.[42] We'll also look at why it can feel so hard to step out of our stress mode. I hope that understanding the evolution of stress in our culture may help you create more calm in your life. I want to start by looking at a bit of history, at the stress that arose when our culture transitioned from hunting-gathering to agriculture and the accumulation of surplus. I want to share a personal experience.

For four years in the early 1990's I served as a pastor for Our Savior's Lutheran church in Nome, Alaska. Half of the people in the congregation came from the Inupiat hunting-gathering tradition. The other half came to Nome from various places in the Lower 48 states, members of the agricultural tradition that started about ten- to twelve-thousand years ago.

Anthropologists write about the huge social and psychological changes that began when we started growing crops rather than hunting game. And since we have only come 10,000 years into this change, it is believed that our genes haven't yet caught up to our new environment. This is part of why we experience a lot of stress – our brain structure and body function haven't adapted yet to the pace and structure that has evolved in our modern world.

For the many hundreds of thousands of years before agriculture, hunting-gathering cultures apparently functioned quite similarly all around the world, small groups of sixty to a few hundred people living together. Cooperation, yes, cooperation, provided the single central organizing feature of these groups. Cooperation, didn't just sound nice, it functioned as the most basic and primary method of survival.

With agriculture came the ability to produce surplus food and then to store that food for long term use. Growing and storing food was new and different from daily foraging.

Once surpluses started accumulating, the game of acquiring and controlling resources transformed our world.

Writing and arithmetic developed as a way to keep records and trade surpluses. Food storage allowed people to develop all sorts of other surpluses, from art works to weapons, and from vacation homes to cellphones. Surplus changed our world away from sharing and cooperation. In its place we came more and more to value acquisition and the competition for resources. Surplus changed our world from calm cooperation to stressful competition. I learned this lesson first-hand while living in Alaska.

One summer while I lived in Nome, two young children each caught their first fish. The memory of those two children and how they handled their first fish has returned to my awareness many times in the years since living in Nome. During that summer long ago, I never imagined the connection to physical health.

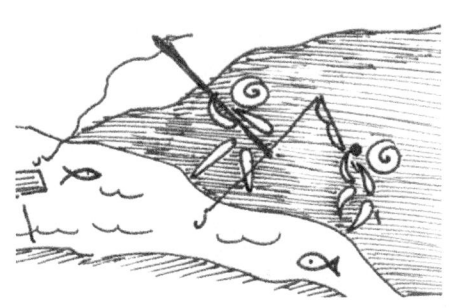

The parents of the one child invited friends for a feast and a celebration. The salmon was prepared and set in front of the little girl. She was served the first piece. We all remarked on her catch and congratulated her.

The little girl's family came from the Lower 48, from the agricultural tradition which started some 10,000 years ago and now dominates the globe.

A little Inupiat boy caught the other first fish. When he came home with his fish he walked it over to his grandmother's house. He gave it to her at the door and then returned home. Grandmother cooked and ate the fish, saving a taste for when her grandson returned to visit.

The little boy followed the Inupiat Eskimo tradition, one of the last vestiges of the hunting-gathering tradition that existed worldwide for hundreds of thousands of years before agriculture became dominant.

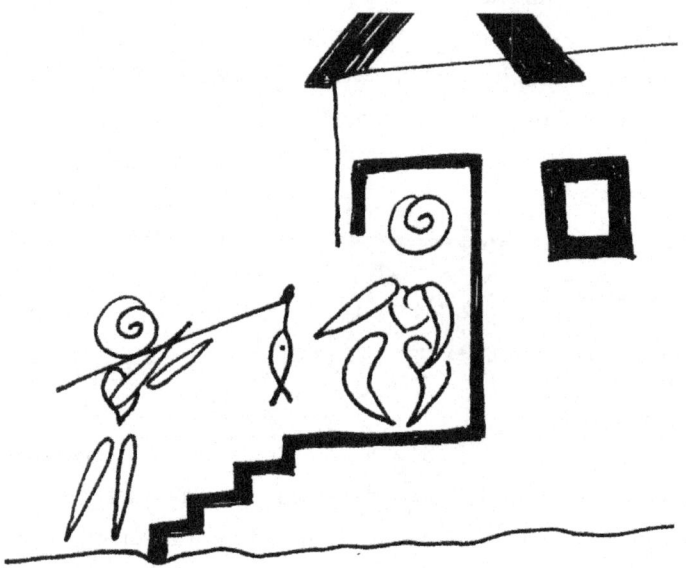

When the little girl got her fish, it was understood from a different framework, from the terms of our modern world - she had acquired a surplus. She was celebrated for that surplus, she got a nice party, and she got the first piece of that surplus. It all happened pretty automatically, and I enjoyed my invitation to this party without giving it any deep thought at the time.

As we discussed earlier, emotions create peptides and peptides glue memories together. The little girl's first fish created a memory that created a peptide that helped to root her in the agricultural paradigm of life, the life of ownership and the control of surplus.

If the little girl grows up to control a lot of surplus, a lot of money and things, she'll probably experience the stress of dealing with her wealth, growing it and managing it, sharing it and defending it and passing it on. Alternatively, if she grows up without enough surplus she'll have stress about the lack and the want in her life. Either way, this little girl is growing up in a world of competition and stress. Academics create grade competition, capitalism promotes economic competition, nationalism tends toward global competition, and even conventional biology promotes the fundamental vision that life itself is a competition where only the fittest survive. When you spend your life competing for stuff and for survival, you get stress. And stress causes the results that make you more likely to go to the doctor.

It wasn't always this way. The hunting-gathering way of cooperation was not just an idealized fantasy, but a fundamental approach to survival that had worked for the hundreds of thousands of years before agriculture and surpluses began. As noted anthropologist Jared Diamond writes, "Hunter-gatherers practiced the most successful and longest-lasting life style in human history. In contrast, we're still struggling with the mess into which agriculture has tumbled us, and it's unclear whether we can solve it."[43]

The little boy who gave the fish to his grandmother grew up in a tradition not focused on accumulating stuff for himself. Hard to believe from our perspective, but this way of sharing was once fundamentally true. The Inupiat traditions are now in a life and death struggle with the power of modern agricultural dominance, but this little boy still learned the way of the old traditions of his culture. When this little boy acquired his surplus, his fish, he knew before he caught it that he would give it away. In his Inupiat tradition he grew up immersed in a way of life that did not focus on accumulating surplus. His way of life evolved to sustain community through cooperation. In sub-arctic Nome, life could not revolve around being an individual in separation from others.

People died in isolation they survived by cooperation.

In times gone by small bands of sixty to a few hundred Inupiat lived in small villages throughout long winters. A person would literally freeze or starve to death if they left their community. More than just a nice idea, life in traditional hunting-gathering society could only continue because cooperation happened automatically as the most basic way of life.

How does this matter to your fibromyalgia pain? If your survival depends on cooperation rather than acquisition, you get a different culture, a less stressed community than what we live in today. If sharing formed the basis of our survival then the stress of competition would diminish and we would have less fight-or-flight response, less autoimmune disease, less fibromyalgia pain. In our society where our language includes competition and "survival of the fittest," as well as "winners and losers," our bodies suffer stress from the get-go, from the very way we have set up our culture.

The way of cooperation apparently guided almost all hunting-gathering cultures before the advent of agricultural surpluses. Once surpluses began to accumulate they snowballed. We now live in the fastest paced, highest technology, most resource intensive environment ever experienced on our planet. We communicate worldwide in instant real time. We work more jobs and more hours than our parents did. We eat genetically modified food whose genes have even been patented and are now sold for profit. For the first time we are now creating human-caused ecological harm on a scale affecting the entire planet.

In our modern world of accelerating surpluses and stresses, how can we be healthy?

First, we're not going back to a true hunting-gathering way of life. You couldn't even choose to do this individually because hunting-gathering is about community – small communities fundamentally committed to the way of cooperation. In many hunting-gathering communities the people were so actively against competition that when a hunter brought back a kill, the rest of the tribe would ridicule the hunter's catch. The tribe had to make sure the hunter didn't start thinking he was anything special or different from the rest of the community. Cooperation was the fundamental asset of these hunting-gathering cultures. In our world, where profitability and competition form the basis of almost every exchange, cooperation is understood differently.

If we can't go back to hunting-gathering, the next best thing might be to increase our awareness about the dynamics of competition. When we understand the source of a stress, we have a better chance of choosing a calm alternative. It's a little like taking off sunglasses and squinting from the sun. When the glasses were on we weren't even aware of their effect. When we took them off we noticed the change, the brightness of the sun. I expect most of us live in this culture of competition without being aware of how completely it dominates our way of life and impacts our health.

As you look at your world without the sunglasses, you can start seeing more and more places where competition dominates. If you consider that every form of competition puts your system on guard (something to win, something to lose) it starts making sense how much stress happens just by living our daily lives.

One thing that will help you is to use The ICE Method every time you notice a stress. This is part of having calm become your default state. As soon as you realize that stress is not from an immediate physical threat you can use The ICE Method and give your body the signal it can return to its calm state. You can do this even in the midst of all your daily stresses. As long as there is no immediate true physical threat, you can shut your fight-or-flight response off again. You can hold internal calm in your life even when surrounded by the winning and losing of a competitive environment.

Using The ICE Method will make a big difference in your life. Awareness will make a difference as well. As you become aware of the ways that competition impacts your life, you may find that this knowledge allows you to create and choose calm alternatives.

Becoming aware of how competition dominates our daily lives can help keep us open to alternatives. If you can change the pattern of your living to more cooperation and less competition, you will put less fight-or-flight stress on your body.

Some years ago, before I knew anything about peptides or The ICE Method, I helped start a community garden. We're a dozen people who garden a half-acre of land together. At the time I was interested in growing local food. What I've come to realize is that I'm growing calm peptides at the same time. I still buy plenty of food from the profit-driven supermarket, but when I participate in the garden and observe plants growing I feel the cooperation of sun, soil, water and plants in nature. When I interact with the other people who are committed to this garden I experience cooperation and I know the stress level is less than many of the other places we spend our time. A community garden might not sound like much in the face of the busy lives we face. Maybe it really isn't much. But it does provide our members one way to experience an alternative to the stress of competition. When we have our hands in soil we have a different perspective - for a moment we have stepped outside of the competitive world that surrounds us. I started this small-scale farming before I knew that it affected my peptide production. Now I know that when I'm in the garden I'm producing more calm peptides: I'm producing the chemistry of health.

I'm not recommending you specifically take up gardening. I do suggest you stay awake and aware for calmer ways to live with the stuff and the stresses of this competitive world. Maybe it's a walk outside, maybe coffee with a friend, perhaps a meditation routine or yoga, or a worship community. However you spend your days, remembering to use The ICE Method for any stress responses will bring you back to your default calm state.

11 - Attachments and Peptides

As I described in the last chapter, I believe cooperation and connection improve health by reduce stress. Those who cooperate and those who feel connected have less that isolates them and less to defend.

An attachment to possessions diminishes health, because whatever I possess you do not possess. The more I possess, the more I must defend, the more I must stress about. One must react against others to control a possession.

Admitting that competition and acquisition have a health cost runs counter to everything we've been taught in our culture – more income is good, for example, and more degrees are good, more insurance is good, more bedrooms, bathrooms, and garages are good, more retirement is good. Whether from the actual possession or the lack of possessing, when we attach our desires to possession, our health suffers.

The lock on our door would make no sense in a traditional Inupiat village. Taking the key out of the car's ignition would be a waste of time. Having a car alarm would be ludicrous. We create our world from our emotions. The emotions associated with possession and isolation help to create stresses and impair our health.

No possession occurs until we first hold a desire in our mind, until we create an emotional peptide that binds together the synapse of a memory and creates "Red Corvette" as a goal. Thirty-three hundred pounds of sports car ends up in our garage because we first held a weightless longing for it.

Your thought weighs nothing, and yet that weightless thought has the power to create a peptide that does have measurable mass. It appears that something gets created from nothing.

Peptides occupy the intersection between what does and what does not exist according to our measurable world.

Peptides have molecular mass so they exist in the world of matter that we can see and weigh. Yet these peptides are formed from a thing which weighs nothing – our emotions.

Change the emotion that has zero weight, and you change the peptide that has a physical mass and weight. Change the emotion; change the health.

Modern Western medicine has focused our attention on this body we can see and measure and weigh. Yet the thing which weighs nothing, our consciousness and emotion, directs the visible body.

Attachments and Peptides

An example - two children suffer bullying at school. One comes home and his parent barks he doesn't want a wimp for a son. As the child cries in confusion and shame, emotions turn to peptides and store in the synapses of the forming memory. The other child comes home to a grandmother and her kitchen table with the warm cookies and hot cocoa. "Tell me," she says, the warmth of love creates different emotional peptides to fill the synapses of the forming memory.

We know from the process and the science of The ICE Method that changing peptides can change our health. When we shift our emotional state to calm and create calm peptides, we free our body to enter a resting and healing state. The thing which weighs nothing can improve the health of our body. When we reconsolidate old traumatic memories and replace the emotional peptides with calm, we lower our body's reactivity and stress. The thing which weighs nothing can transform the fear, anger, and other distress that stored for so long in our bodies.

When we access the space that holds nothing, the space of calm, we feel better. When we find ourselves stuck reacting to distressed emotions about people, places, things and ideas, then we use up our body's energy on external reactions instead of internal rest and healing. Distress drains our ability to heal.

During my time as a pastor in Nome, I observed something that I now understand as memory reconsolidation. Sometime before I arrived, in a fit of drunkenness, one night a young man shot and killed his wife. The father of the husband and the father of the wife had been good friends before the tragedy. In this church where I served the members had a tradition of singing solos or group songs to mark special occasions. One day, a couple years after the tragedy, these two fathers walked together up the aisle to the front of the church. Side by side they stood before the congregation and sang together in their native language. Everyone had on their mind the terrible tragedy as these two men sang. The singing and the love and the forgiveness of these two fathers also created a different state with different peptide molecules to reconsolidate the memory of the tragedy. Cooperation at this level tends toward calm and peace and health for a whole community.

The ICE Method provides a powerful option for stepping back from the stressed entanglement of possessions, control, and isolation. The ICE Method gives you a process for being in the state of calm and peace. The ICE Method also employs memory reconsolidation in order to replace accumulated stresses from the past so you can stay in the state of calm. Once you start using The ICE Method and start experiencing better health, you may feel a lightness developing about your attachment to the stuff and the stresses of this world. You may feel you have less to defend. You may feel more peace coming to your spirit.

If you have suffered the symptoms of fibromyalgia, it may have consumed most of your energy. Once you start feeling better, you may start asking questions. What is my good health for? What is my purpose? What am I here for? For the sake of improving your health, I believe it's important to pay attention to cooperation and belonging. More possessions and more control are not likely to heal your body. Health has to do with the wholeness of your spirit.

Historically, religions have been one of the ways we converse about things that matter. I thought hard about this, but finally decided to include a few words about religion. If religion has caused you more stress than peace, you can read or ignore these words as you wish. As a former pastor I've probably seen religions cause more damage than most people could imagine. And yet, I also appreciate that at their best, religions have made some important contributions to the conversations about living well in our world. Hopefully, these words can offer one more piece in helping your fibromyalgia symptoms get better and stay better.

The world's great religions of Judaism, Hinduism, Buddhism, Christianity, and Islam all evolved long after the establishment of agriculture. I have come to believe that world religions developed to remind us what we lost when we shifted away from the cooperation of hunting and gathering. I believe the major world religions arose as a response to the problems of surplus. They tell us to share and love, because these ancient hunting-gathering essentials were being lost to the competition and acquisition of agriculture. If our religions are talking about surplus, then perhaps they can help us live with more cooperation and a greater sense of belonging. Perhaps they can provide us with insights for our health.

Let me start with Buddhism and Hinduism. These two traditions offer direct encouragement for recovering the hunting-gatherers non-attachment to your first fish or any other possessions. The Buddha said simply, "Free yourself from attachment." In the freedom from attachment we grow our ability to reduce suffering and increase happiness. From the perspective of hunting and gathering, the Buddha's encouragement feels similar to the mindset of a cooperative community. Hunter-gatherers don't acquire anything for their own sake, but for the well-being of the whole community. From the perspective of peptides and memory reconsolidation, non-attachment produces a calm state. In the state of calm, the peptides of anger and fear do not store in our bodies. When we have calm, when we have non-attachment, we can be present and aware, rather than reactive and disturbed.

In Judaism, the book of Genesis begins with two differing versions of Adam and Eve in the Garden of Eden. In the second of these stories, Adam and Eve get to name all the plants and animals. Comparing to the Buddha's words about non-attachment, the naming of the plants and animals already begins creating attachments – if you name something you are closer to controlling and owning it. When Adam and Eve hear they must avoid only one of the trees in the garden, they quickly begin to desire that too. As they become attached to possessing the apple, they eat the fruit and then God banishes them from the garden. God's description of the agricultural life that follows is not at all pretty: "Cursed is the ground because of you: through painful toil you will eat food from it all the days of your life."

From this point of the Scripture and onwards you could look at the rest of the Jewish teaching as a conversation about how to live in the world as it transitions from hunting and gathering to agriculture and surpluses. How can the Jewish people share the goods amongst themselves? How shall kings govern? How can the nation fight or have peace with other nations? How will surplus be distributed? The Adam and Eve story described the transition from the non-attachment of hunting and gathering to the toil for acquiring the surplus and possessions of agriculture. Scholars who study the message of the Jewish Scriptures often comment on how consistently the texts command hospitality to strangers along with faithfulness to their God. We are meant for cooperation and sharing. The Jewish faith encourages people to remember this truth.

Jesus lived his life as a person of the Jewish faith. His teachings formed the basis of Christianity and he too consistently addressed the problems of attaching to our stuff. He is famous for telling people to give their possessions to the poor and then to come and follow him. In another episode, in the Fourth chapter of Matthew, Jesus undergoes temptation in the wilderness.

After Jesus survives the forty days, then he is tempted by the devil who offers stones that can become bread for him, power that can be his, and the kingdoms of the world he can control. It's a telling story – Jesus faces the temptations of surplus, yet he deliberately chooses to stay non-attached to the possessions, the control and the power of this world.

In our world where ownership is so important, Jesus word's often come across as an affront to our way of living. I believe, though, that Jesus was offering us a way of non-attachment, a way of freedom. Ultimately, being less concerned about how much we own, or how well we compare with others, will free us to enjoy better health.

In our society, making the choice to share and cooperate requires a deliberate and counter-cultural choice. We teach sharing to our kids, but what we observe and what we do in daily life often contradicts; getting the best grade in school, getting into the most prestigious college, the profit-maximizing of corporations, the warring of nations, and the advertisements that stoke our cravings. We teach sharing in a world that operates on isolation, acquisition, competition and the survival of the fittest. This is one of the reasons I chose to include this reflection on religion. In the competition-based world we live in, anything that helps us develop a lightness toward our stuff will help improve our health.

Attachments and Peptides

Modern New Age and self-help approaches have flourished, perhaps to add answers for how we might live in this world of surplus. Some modern approaches promise spiritual techniques so we can acquire more riches. These are fundamentally opposite to the approaches that help people see the value of non-attachment. *A Course in Miracles* is one example of the many that point toward non-attachment. Its program focuses completely on developing a different view of physical things so we can recognize an unfailing truth: We are One with the source of all life and we are One with humanity. *A Course in Miracles* goes so far in this direction that it claims our world is but an illusion whose sole purpose is to help us recognize that we are already One with the source. Believing we can be separate from the source and from others is the illusion. We live to wake up from this illusion. Our purpose is to become aware of the only true thing – that all of us are equally and fully connected to the ultimate source and to each other, forever and ever. *A Course in Miracles*, and other similar approaches are about as opposite as one can imagine to the "survival of the fittest" mentality of our modern world.

In hunting-gathering cultures, the attachment to community and the non-attachment to material wealth were not choices to be made in opposition to the culture. Instead, cooperation and sharing were the essence of the culture. Hunter-gatherers didn't need the to view the material world as an illusion in order to develop non-attachment. They passed on the value of sharing because it provided survival value. The little boy who caught his fish and gave it to his grandmother did it so he could survive. He simply did what had made this way of living thrive for hundreds of thousands of years.

Developing non-attachment lightens our worry about competition and about stuff. Non-attachment can also increase a sense of connection with others and all that exists. As the isolating influence of our attachments decreases, a sense for the innate equality and sacredness of all people may arise in its place. In such a space of calm, the body fears no enemy, and seeks no angry actions. The body moves into a state of rest, healing, and restoration.

The ICE Method came about as I followed the question, "how do we heal?" The ICE Method didn't arise out of any religious background or worldviews; it arose to help individuals heal. As I watched people go through the experience of becoming pain free I became more and more aware of how much our physical bodies exist as a product of our stored emotional histories. I also observed that our health relates to the spirit we bring to living in the world. I feel thankful to have become aware that entering the calm space and exchanging peptides can put us on the road to emotional freedom and spiritual peace. If we take the example of hunter-gatherers, healing happens not just for the individual, but also for the clan we belong to.

Attachments and Peptides

Today, our clan now includes the entire planet. Our healing includes the whole world. It turns out that our most modern science confirms our connections and the value of compassion more deeply than any of us may have ever imagined. Scientific understanding has transformed from "survival of the fittest" to a complete interconnection of everything in the universe across all time and all space. Amazingly, modern science has extended the religious understanding of "love" to include everything, everywhere, and for all time. Modern science confirms that each and every one of us is an essential part of this whole universe. Getting a taste for this modern quantum science might be more than just interesting – this way of understanding may provide yet another avenue for you to embrace calm in your life and have fewer symptoms of fibromyalgia. We'll take a closer look at this in the next chapter.

12 - Energy and Matter

You probably started this book because of the pain you experienced from fibromyalgia. If you have had significant symptoms, you may have lived as a servant to the pain. If you were like those with more severe cases of fibromyalgia you couldn't dependably keep a calendar, because you never knew when your body would or would not function without excruciating pain. Your body controlled your life.

In *Fibromyalgia Relief* we have opened up a method that allows us to live from a different perspective on truth:

**body follows mind, and our
fight-or-flight system can be turned off.**

Hopefully your pain has begun or will soon begin to subside as you apply The ICE Method to your life. Learning The ICE Method provides a way to reduce personal stress, which often leads to a decrease or elimination of fibromyalgia and other chronic pains.

Unfortunately, unless a person continues to pay conscious attention, returning to one's old familiar environment can cause a renewal of stress and the return of pain.

We need to choose to stay aware.

A person who wants to stay better will benefit by continuing to pay attention whenever anything arises that does not feel calm. As long as the upset doesn't cause a true immediate physical danger, the stress can be taken out of the situation right then by using The ICE method. Use this on memories and emotions as they arise and ensure they reconsolidate. Part One focused on this process, the steps and the science of The ICE Method.

After learning the technique of The ICE Method our focus switched to gaining some cultural and religious, perspectives on sharing, compassion, calm and health. My goal was to add some background so you can begin to live less reactively to this surplus-oriented world. If you begin seeing how profoundly our world changed as agricultural surpluses started to accumulate, then you also begin seeing the underlying reasons for so much of our personal and societal suffering. The great religions addressed these questions and recommended that developing non-attachment to the things of this material world could increase our satisfaction and our sense of connectedness with others.

Now I want to look at how our most modern science, quantum mechanics, supports an understanding of our universal connectedness at the deepest levels of our consciousness and our being.

The old Newtonian science of the physical world and Darwin's theory of the "survival of the fittest" fit well with our worldview as it grew more and more centered on controlling the material world. Yet, now even that old science has begun moving on. For the past hundred years quantum mechanics has explored the action of subatomic particles. It turns out that on the quantum level: what you see depends on how you look at it.

The way you observe is important in quantum mechanics, and it's also a perfect description of how The ICE Method relieves your fibromyalgia symptoms. If you live with fibromyalgia from a state of fight-or flight you get a different result than living out of a state of calm. Understanding the perspective of quantum mechanics could well help you feel better.

In the quantum world, scientists observe that matter really does follow mind. Scientists have performed countless experiments to verify what is called the observer effect. How a scientist chooses to observe an experiment affects what will show up in the experimental results. In terms of The ICE Method, we see all the time that body follows mind. Change your mind from stress to calm, and you will change your body.

In the quantum world scientists relate matter to energy by Einstein's famous equation, $E = mc^2$. Matter and energy are directly connected. It turns out, though, that even when you remove all available energy from a given space, there's still more energy in it, a fluctuating intersection between energy and the momentary flashes of particles called the Zero Point Field. In this quantum field every piece of energy is connected. If something happens at one place in the Zero Point Field, the effects show up instantaneously throughout the field. Strange but true in the quantum worldview.

This Zero Point Field is apparently present everywhere throughout the universe. It's quite literally mind-boggling. Get this - a cubic meter, less than the space under your dining room table, contains enough energy to boil all the oceans of the world.[44] And because waves also store information as well as transmit energy, scientists believe that all the information of all the books stored in the Library of Congress could be contained in the Zero Point Field in a space the size of a sugar cube. This information is available throughout the field, everywhere and instantaneously. It's way too much for me to grasp, but just a few perceptions about quantum can be enough to transform our perceptions about this material life.

In the quantum world scientists think of vibrations instead of material things. In quantum, the explanation would use waves instead of peptides, but The ICE Method makes sense either way. Peptides are what show up in the concrete material visible world, but they originate as a result of consciousness, of information, of emotion. Peptides are the material result of emotions

Energy and Matter

and the Zero Point Field. Emotional peptides come from this vast universal field of inconceivable energy and incredible information.

There's another word for this - scientists call the phenomenon of connection, entanglement. It becomes impossible to fully separate out any single thing from the whole. One particle affects another. Change the one and the other responds. Repeated experiments have confirmed this entanglement property of quantum mechanics. Things get shared in the quantum world. The quantum world is more like the sharing of a hunting-gathering culture, it's a cooperating, entangled universe.

Scientists once believed that nothing travels faster than the speed of light. Now we know that information is not limited by the speed of light; it can transmit instantaneously. Information can affect physical objects such as electrons without any delay of time. Even the past, present, and future are all entangled. This helps us understand how exchanging the peptides of a decades-old upset can sometimes bring almost instant healing in the present experience of our bodily health.

A challenge for researchers has been taking findings on the subatomic level and applying them to the level of living organisms and bigger objects. Most quantum researchers, in fact, limit themselves to the subatomic world where they can more easily observe quantum effects. Some scientists, though, do look for how quantum physics operates on the larger physical level. One person who did just this is Fritz Albert Popp.[45] As far back as the 1970's, he had already discovered that living beings emit light waves. He measured this light in the form of tiny quantum behaving photons. He discovered that in healthy humans this light was entangled and coherent – it carried information. The light we emit comes from interaction with the Zero Point Field. This, believes Popp, provides the answer even for how our bodies take shape from conception and how we become who we are. Our biology exists in a direct relationship to the quantum field. Traditional biologists haven't been able to find a chemical or electrical answer for how the body can coordinate 50-100 trillion cells each undergoing something like 100,000 chemical reactions per second. Quantum entanglement offers an explanation consistent with this amazing coordination of the cells of our bodies and minds.

In further tests, Popp explored the relationship between the light emitted and a person's health. He compared the light emitted by healthy people to people with cancer and people with Multiple Sclerosis. Compared to healthy people, cancer sufferers emitted less light. In their suffering from cancer, they had too little light (too little information) in their bodies to coordinate healthy cellular activity. One can imagine that without proper coordination, cells could begin to grow haphazardly without the necessary healthy template of information being provided by the light waves. It is believed that this is just what happens in the development of cancer cells.

In Multiple Sclerosis, it turns out that people take in and emit more light (more information) than healthy people. In MS, when people take in too much light it corresponds to taking in too much organization and control. This light is also less coherent, less patterned, more disturbed. As the body accepts too much confused information from its external environment it restricts the body's systems with too many instructions so the body cannot freely maintain health. Interestingly for our concern with fibromyalgia, Multiple Sclerosis is listed as an autoimmune disorder. In autoimmunity, internal stress and a stuck fight-or-flight response have turned the body's immune system against itself. Popp's studies of stress confirmed that a person's light emission rises when they experience stress. In chronic autoimmunity terms, the body has lost its ability to distinguish between external and internal threat, the body has lost its freedom to react appropriately to the environment. In terms of quantum light, the body is absorbing too much light, too much information, too many conditions, too many constraints. It would make sense that one of the autoimmune characteristics is inflammation, the body's reaction to bombardment by the external environment, by the quantum field.

Quantum changes our scientific worldview from isolation and separation to entanglement and infinite cooperation. In the quantum world we humans, just like subatomic particles, are also pure energy, and pure information. We are connected to past and future as much as to this present moment. What we observe in this material moment of our existence is a function of our consciousness, of the way that we observe.

If we allow ourselves to embrace this quantum understanding, we can envision our material lives unfolding as a direct result of our consciousness. The ICE Method is consistent with this quantum understanding – body follows mind. Consciousness creates our experience in this material world. Isolation, separateness, individuality are all illusion. Pay attention to your mind and your energy. Your body follows your mind.

How often have we been advised to take care of ourselves, and we just end up feeling more stressed by how huge the self-care job feels? The ICE Method provides a much simpler way to pay attention to your mind and body. The process is consistent all the way from spiritual understandings to chemistry to quantum. But you do have to show up for it.

You have to bring your consciousness to health.

If you do, The ICE Method provides a direct process for truly interacting with your health on the physical, emotional, and spiritual levels.

The ICE Method focuses on changing peptides in our body and brain. I believe that in the calm space, when we stop being reactive to these material peptides, we find ourselves able to access the information and the waves. It is believed that this is just what happens in the development of cancer cells.

In Multiple Sclerosis, it turns out that people take in and emit more light (more information) than healthy people. In MS, when people take in too much light it corresponds to taking in too much organization and control. This light is also less coherent, less patterned, more disturbed. As the body accepts too much confused information from its external environment it restricts the body's systems with too many instructions so the body cannot freely maintain health. Interestingly for our concern with fibromyalgia, Multiple Sclerosis is listed as an autoimmune disorder. In autoimmunity, internal stress and a stuck fight-or-flight response have turned the body's immune system against itself. Popp's studies of stress confirmed that a person's light emission rises when they experience stress. In chronic autoimmunity terms, the body has lost its ability to distinguish between external and internal threat, the body has lost its freedom to react appropriately to the environment. In terms of quantum light, the body is absorbing too much light, too much information, too many conditions, too many constraints. It would make sense that one of the autoimmune characteristics is inflammation, the body's reaction to bombardment by the external environment, by the quantum field.

Quantum changes our scientific worldview from isolation and separation to entanglement and infinite cooperation. In the quantum world we humans, just like subatomic particles, are also pure energy, and pure information. We are connected to past and future as much as to this present moment. What we observe in this material moment of our existence is a function of our consciousness, of the way that we observe.

If we allow ourselves to embrace this quantum understanding, we can envision our material lives unfolding as a direct result of our consciousness. The ICE Method is consistent with this quantum understanding – body follows mind. Consciousness creates our experience in this material world. Isolation, separateness, individuality are all illusion. Pay attention to your mind and your energy. Your body follows your mind.

How often have we been advised to take care of ourselves, and we just end up feeling more stressed by how huge the self-care job feels? The ICE Method provides a much simpler way to pay attention to your mind and body. The process is consistent all the way from spiritual understandings to chemistry to quantum. But you do have to show up for it.

You have to bring your consciousness to health.

If you do, The ICE Method provides a direct process for truly interacting with your health on the physical, emotional, and spiritual levels.

The ICE Method focuses on changing peptides in our body and brain. I believe that in the calm space, when we stop being reactive to these material peptides, we find ourselves able to access the information and the energy of the Zero Point Field. The ICE Method, by helping you enter the calm state, helps you move into a coherent light and energy state. As Lynne McTaggart phrases it in *The Field*:

> Health is a state of perfect subatomic communication, and ill health is a state where communication breaks down. We are ill when our waves are out of synch.[46]

I also believe that quantum mechanics offers a powerful expression of freedom, of non-attachment. After 10,000 years of playing the agricultural material surplus game, our best understanding of the world is returning to a much more ancient understanding, that our conscious energy describes who we are. It turns out that quantum theory coincides much better with the way of cooperation followed by hunting-gathering societies. Quantum also matches the traditions of the great world religions, in their advocacy for non-attachment and for loving our neighbor as our self. Energy or spirit provides a better explanation than pure materialism. If quantum mechanics applies on our human scale as well as on the subatomic scale, then we are all "entangled," connected, related. If this is true, then quantum entanglement offers a better description than competition and survival of the fittest. It doesn't even make sense for us to remain rigidly attached to the way we observe a situation, because with each observation we change it.

Think again about our fight-or-flight mechanism. When fight-or-flight gets stuck, it keeps us glued in reaction mode to the threats of this material world. With a consciousness of fight-or-flight stuck ON, we can only react with fear or anger. When we sense danger, our fight-or-flight consciousness results in literal material peptides that limit us to reacting with fear or anger. Creating stress, these peptides that govern our actions also impact our health.

Our consciousness shapes our experience of health.

The ICE Method, using memory reconsolidation, gives us a technique for consciously changing our emotional history. The ICE Method is a tool that lets us bridge the past, present, and future. As we replace material peptides of old memories or future fears, we change our consciousness and material expression of our present lives. We go from stressed responses to calm. In this change of viewpoint, our material health responds and shows up as a reflection of calm. Entering the calm state creates changes in a person's experience of health and well-being.

Quantum understanding provides an even more basic understanding than the peptide explanation for how The ICE Method works. Quantum also provides a more direct correlation to the non-attachment emphases of hunting-gathering culture and the great world religions of the agricultural world; Hinduism,

Buddhism, Judaism, Christianity, and Islam. I've chosen to explain The ICE Method in terms of material peptides because I've found that most of us can more easily imagine peptide molecules than quantum mechanical vibrations. Peptides are the first thing that shows up in our material body once we have a conscious experience, so they are directly connected to this quantum understanding. Peptides are also measurable. Once you get a feel for exchanging peptides, the process is simple and direct. Extraordinary effects can result when a peptide exchange process is used. Quantum understanding can expand your understanding and appreciation, but on its own, The ICE Method keeps the images simple.

For healing to last, one must learn to shut off the fight-or-flight response and to keep it turned off. I have included these brief words on hunting-gathering and religions and quantum because I believe that for our fight-or-flight response to turn off and stay off we must ultimately come to believe we are safe in this world. We must learn that we have something meaningful to offer to the experience of living. Ironically, non-attachment has a much better record for making us feel safe than stuff, possession, and control.

At its core, the fight-or-flight response is a physical thing, a certain arrangement of stuff called amino acids stacked together in a peptide molecule, all of which first showed up in response to consciousness. When we live attached to the chemistry of our fight-or-flight response, our health suffers. When our self-concept grows instead to understand we are not limited by time and space, our experience of life grows fuller. When we realize our material bodies are grounded in energy that includes an everlasting flow of the past, present, and future, then it gets easier for us to see we are all equal partners in this experience of humanity. When we understand that the universe is both entangled and cooperative, we can see how living more harmoniously provides deep satisfaction and improvements to our health. Length of life becomes less critical: Quality of life grows more treasured. We come to recognize that the quality of all life is inextricably woven together in an entangled field of what the great traditions call love. From this place we enjoy the consciousness and the material expression of health and wholeness.

13 – The ICE Method

I believe that having a simple tool such as The ICE Method can help you feel better. I have kept this book short because my focus is on giving you a usable tool. In fact, just reading Chapters One, Three, and Five will give you the technique for calming emotions and replacing peptides. The other chapters of Part One provide the science behind the method. If you have read only the technique chapters from this book – I hope you discovered a valuable tool. It's a tool for your entire life – whenever non-calm arises, you have a simple way to restore calm to your life.

For those of you who think a lot about health and wellness, I have provided my understanding of the chemistry, the anthropology, the religious perspective and the quantum understanding to hopefully help you see that reducing or eliminating your fibromyalgia pain makes good sense. Health, in my opinion, and as my deep wish, should be our common experience.

As best as I can understand, The ICE Method is consistent with both ancient traditions and modern science as a tool for growing your health and wholeness. If your interest is like mine you'll be searching the Internet and devouring books, engaged in growing your experience of health and life.

As I have written this book, I have remained acutely aware of my lack of a medical credential or a degree in biology. Despite a physician friend of mine who keeps reminding me I have a science degree in engineering and also a degree in divinity studies, I still feel like an intruder into the field of Western medical health. Like most people I grew up believing my health was in the hands of doctors. As I work with more and more people, I grow increasingly aware of how different The ICE Method is from modern medical practice. Who am I to write a book on health?

This is what I've come up with.

> Estimates vary from four to fifteen million people who suffer from the symptoms of fibromyalgia in the United States, and millions more worldwide.

> The current Western medical system of treatment does not work well for most of these people, yet standard medical treatment costs an enormous amount of money and energy.

> The ICE Method actually does provide strong results for many people, and for very little money – either the price of this book, membership in the MyFibromyalgiaRelief community, or at most some personal sessions with an experienced person.

Fibromyalgia Relief is what I have to offer to the conversation of reducing the suffering caused by fibromyalgia. Read the disclaimer and use this resource in whatever ways you find most helpful.

In writing this book, I have used The ICE Method and this process of reconsolidating old peptides as my own fears have arisen about possible reactions to The ICE Method. I imagine all sorts of professional critiques of this book: where are the studies, the long term results, the brain scan tests to confirm what the calm state looks like using brain imaging techniques? Why haven't you waited until you worked with 1,000 people instead of just 100? None of those critiques could cause me immediate physical harm. So, I use The ICE Method on them. And yet, I do hope for critiques that arrive with goodwill so we can find answers and grow the usefulness of The ICE Method or replace it with something even better.

For whatever reason, I have been fortunate enough to become aware of this ICE Method process. I have seen this process transform lives. I have grown to believe deeply in this process. And when I see other processes that also work I can usually see how memory reconsolidation is taking place as the primary causative factor in those techniques.

I want you and anyone else with fibromyalgia to have access to The ICE Method or any other method that can help you to feel well. I want the suffering from fibromyalgia to stop. As I said at the beginning of this book, I haven't discovered anything new, although the scientific understanding of memory reconsolidation is itself a recent discovery. If there's anything new here it's the combination of insights into a simple method that provides quick results and the possibility of turning off a person's fight-or-flight response for good.

So, here you have it, The ICE Method for relieving or eliminating your symptoms of fibromyalgia. It comes with my best wishes that fibromyalgia can be reduced as a cause of suffering in your life and in our wide world.

May you live calm.

Thank you, and best wishes,

Lars Clausen

Epilogue: A Review

People who suffer from fibromyalgia typically have their fight-or-flight stress response stuck in the ON position. This stresses the body and results in symptoms. If the fight-or-flight response can be turned off, then symptoms will diminish or disappear.

To turn off the fight-of-flight response you can use The ICE Method to enter a calm state and create a different chemistry for your body. **Identify. Calm. Exchange.**

Observe a single point. Since this is a simple task for your mind, your body begins to relax. *Body Follows Mind.*

Observe a second point. The body continues to relax

Observe the empty space between the two points. When you do this your mind signals your body that there is nothing in the external environment that needs a response. Peptides are created that correspond to this calm state and your body responds with calm. Your fight-or-flight response turns off.

ICE: To calm the emotions of stored memories use the ICE Method to exchange peptides.

1. **Identify the stored emotion** to activate the stored peptides. Notice emotions, memories, and physical sensations.

2. **Enter the calm state** and rest in this state for a few moments

3. **Exchange peptides.** Observe the stored emotion again. Notice whatever has changed

Repeat the process until everything that shows up feels calm.

Pursue wholeness: Find some way to develop a sense of wholeness to support your health.

Hunting-Gathering traditions emphasized our connectedness and the survival value of sharing.

Religious traditions reiterated the ancient emphasis on connection and sharing, reminding adherents that God and neighbor offer a more healthy focus than acquisition and competition.

Science, through quantum mechanics, supports the deepest understanding of our innate connectedness with one another and with everything in the universe.

As we use The ICE Method and become calm, we can discover better health and a renewed sense of purpose and belonging for our lives.

Disclaimer:

Lars Clausen is not a medical doctor. He holds a Master's Degree in Mechanical Engineering and earned a Master of Divinity Degree preceding his service as a pastor. Lars Clausen does not offer medical advice. He uses the non-invasive ICE Method to work with people who bring emotional or physical issues for relief. Lars Clausen is not responsible for clients' experience with The ICE Method or their results.

The ICE Method is not traditional Western medicine – it is not medicine. The hypothesis is that the ICE Method works by invoking an awareness of emotional responses engaging neuropeptides in the process of memory reconsolidation. In this process the body and mind will often experience relief. The ICE Method is in an experimental stage. You must use your own common sense in deciding the appropriateness of The ICE Method for you. If you have any medical or other questions about using The ICE Method, you should consult with your health care provider before using The ICE Method or scheduling a session.

The ICE Method does not guarantee either specific or general outcomes for clients. The contents of this book make no guarantee as to accuracy or results. All content is the personal opinion of Lars Clausen and is not medical or psychological advice. Usage of any content is the responsibility of the reader.

Notes:

[1] G. Liptan, Figuring Out Fibromyalgia, (Portland, Oregon, Visceral Press, 2011.)

[2] B. Lipton, The Biology of Belief, (Carlsbad, California, Hay House, 2008.) 115-124.

[3] C. Pert, Molecules of Emotion, (New York, Scribner, 1997.)

Candace Pert continues to do groundbreaking work on the mechanisms of cellular communication and response. Pert has published over 250 scientific papers. Her book, *Molecules of Emotion*, offered a clear presentation of peptides and cellular functioning to those outside of the research community. This book changed the way I understand the human body and is one of the pivotal books that helped me become aware of how we can influence our own healing. Highly recommended.

[4] Pert.

[5] F. Kinslow, The Secret of Instant Healing, (USA, Lucid Sea, 2008.)

[6] Lipton.

[7] B. Ecker, R Ticic, L. Hulley, Unlocking the Emotional Brain, (New York, Routledge, 2012.) 14.

I have followed Ecker's dating of memory reconsolidation. Ecker identifies the 2004 published research of Pedreira, Pérez-Cuesta, and Maldonado as the primary research demonstrating "how to induce reconsolidation behaviorally through a series of experiences required by the brain for erasure." This article is entitled, "Mismatch Between What is Expected and What Actually Occurs Triggers Memory Reconsolidation or Extinction." Earlier work by Karim Nader and others had discovered the process of retrieved memories becoming labile, for example, Nader, Schafe, and LeDoux, "Fear Memories Require Protein Synthesis in the Amygdala for Reconsolidation After Retrieval." Nature, August 2000. Later work by Daniella Schiller demonstrated the reconsolidation process in an experiment using human subjects. Schiller, Monfils, Raio, Johnson, LeDoux, Phelps, "Preventing the Return of Fear in Humans Using Reconsolidation Update Mechanisms." Nature, January, 2010.

[8] Ecker.

[9] Ecker. 14.

[10] Ecker, 202.

[11] D. Schiller, M. Monfils, C Raio, D. Johnson, J LeDoux, E. Phelps, "Preventing the return of fear in humans using reconsolidation update mechanisms," (Nature – Vol 463, Issue 7277 January 7, 2010, doi:10.1038/nature 08637.)

[12] LeDoux, The Synaptic Self: How Our Brains Become Who We Are. (New York, Penguin, 2002). 161

[13] Liptan, 17-20, 105-109.

[14] Pert.

[15] Ecker, 13.

[16] J. Dispenza, Evolve Your Brain, (Deerfield Beach, Florida, 2007.)

[17] Schiller.

[18] Ecker.

[19] L. Watkins, M. Hutchinson, E. Milligan, S. Maier, "Listening" and "talking" to neurons: Implications of immune activation for pain control and increasing the efficacy of opioids" (Brain Res Rev. 2007 November; 56(1): 148–169.)

[20] K. Ren, R. Dubner, "Neuron-glia crosstalk gets serious: Role in pain hypersensitivity." (Curr Opin Anaesthesiol. 2008 October; 21(5): 570–579.)

[21] J. Shah, E. Gilliams, "Uncovering the biochemical milieu of myofascial trigger points using in vivo microdialysis: An application of muscle pain concepts to myofascial pain syndrome." (Journal of Bodywork and Movement Therapies, 2008, 12, 371-384.)

[22] Pert, 168-173.
[23] Pert, 242-243.
[24] Pert, 243.
[25] Watkins.
[26] Watkins.
[27] Shah.
[28] F. Behm, I. Gavin, O Karpenko, V. Lindgren, S Gaitonde, P Gashkoff, B Gillis, "Unique immunological patterns in fibromyalgia." (BMC Clinical Pathology, December, 2012, http://www.biomedcentral.com/1472-6890/12/25.)
[29] R. Tynan, S. Naicker, M. Hinwood, E. Nalivaiko, K. Butler, D. Pow, T. Day, and F. Walker, "Chronic stress alters the density and morphology of microglia in a subset of stress-responsive brain regions," (Brain Behav Immun. 2010 Oct; 24 (7):1058-68. doi: 10.1016/j.bbi.2010.02.001. Epub 2010 Feb 11.)
[30] S. Sugama, T Taknouchi, M Fujita, B. Conti, and M. Hashimoto, "Differential microglial activation between acute stress and lipopolysaccharide treatment." (Journal of Neuroimmunology, V. 207, Issues 1-2, Feb 2009, 24-31.)
[31] N. Uceyler, D. Zeller, A Kahn, S Kewenig, S Kittle-Schneider, A. Schmid, J. Casnova-Molla, K. Reiners, C. Sommer, "Small fibre pathology in patients with fibromyalgia syndrome." (Brain. 2013 Jun;136(Pt 6):1857-67. doi: 10.1093/brain/awt053. Epub 2013 Mar 918.)
[32] A. Oaklander, Report at American Neurological Association, 137th Annual Meeting.
[33] Liptan 28.
[34] Liptan, 56.
[35] G Maté, When The Body Says No, (Hoboken, New Jersey, John Wiley and Sons, 2003).
[36] Maté, 173.
[37] Maté, 175-176.
[38] Maté, 33.
[39] Maté, 35.
[40] J. Ledoux, The Emotional Brain: The Mysterious Underpinnings of Emotional Life, New York, Simon and Schuster, 1996.) 242.
[41] Liptan, 56.

[42] American Pschological Association, "How Does Stress Affect Us?," (http://psychcentral.com/lib/how-does-stress-affect-us/0001130.)

[43] J. Diamond, "The Worst Mistake in the History of the Human Race" (Discover Magazine, May 1987. 64-66.)

[44] L. McTaggart, The Field, (New York, Harper, 2008.) 19.

[45] McTaggart, 39-53.

[46] McTaggart, 52.

Made in the USA
Monee, IL
14 June 2022